LOSE WEIGHT, FEEL GREAT!

EVEN AFTER KIDS

BY
MARY CAROLINE
RHEA

todaysbalanced**mom**.com

LOSE WEIGHT, FEEL GREAT!

© 2011 Mary Caroline Rhea

CreateSpace, a DBA of On-Demand Publishing LLC, part of the Amazon group of companies.

ISBN # 978-1-4348-1671-9

Book & cover design: Steve Lepre/Sunhead Projects, LLC
Photography: Jack Alterman

Printed in the United States of America

DEDICATION

I would like to dedicate this book to my parents, "Bebo" and Douglas Heath, for bringing me up in a home that made eating healthy, exercise and participating in sports a part of our daily lives even before the rest of the world was on the big health kick. During my high school years, my mother and I would rise early enough to meet my aunt, Caroline Reed, and best friend, Harriet Weeks Pollitzer, so we could go for a run before school. My Mom and Aunt Caroline were proud owners of the original waffle baby blue Nike running shoes with the yellow swoosh. This was the first running shoe of its kind, and the first of many to come. Yes, they were right there when the concept of running for fun was a novelty. I will forever be grateful to my Mom who taught me how to water ski at the age of five never once complaining about treading water in the creeks of Charleston as I skied away. I am extremely grateful to my Mom, who always read about health and fitness and was ahead of her time on the importance of a healthy diet and its long term effects.

I also want to thank my Dad for making me my first barbell out of a broom stick and old weights when I was only six years old. My older brother and I would watch out the window waiting for Dad pull in from work, and rush out to greet him so we could "lift weights" and then time each other as we ran sprints around our property. Thank you Dad, for teaching me how to catch, throw and punt a football and all the other sport related skills you shared with me. Thanks for teaching me the things that some dads neglect to teach their daughters.

Thanks to the both of you for giving me the love of staying active and eating healthy!

I would like to give a special thank you to my life long friend, Gready Rowland Frazier. She has been a great supporter of my efforts with this book and with my company. She has spent countless hours helping me with the editing of *Lose Weight, Feel Great!* and I am forever grateful to her.

Thank you to my book designer Steve Lepre who has seen me go through a lot of life changes while trying to get this book in print. Thank you for a wonderful job and for being so fun to work with.

To my husband John, I not only dedicate this book but my life! It started off as being childhood sweethearts at the age of 11, to a blended family of seven boys and then being blessed with our little girl, Mary Ellis!

TABLE OF CONTENTS

Chapter 6:
Creating an Effective Workout Program

Chapter 7:
Simple Tricks to Help You Lose

Chapter 8:
Questions and Answers about Diet and Fitness

Chapter 9:
Easy, Diet-Friendly Recipes for You and Your Family

INTRODUCTION

We all know that being a mom is the most rewarding experience you could ever have. We also know that is doesn't come without a few challenges - most good things do. Creating life is a true miracle but it does leave our bodies with some things to overcome. Just a few of those include (1) the fact that you have the necessary weight gain during pregnancy to get rid of, (2) weight doesn't come off as easily as it use to, (3) our focus is on our family and not ourselves, (4) our time is stretched thin due to the demands of raising a family, and (5) thanks to childbirth those hips just aren't quite the same as they use to be.

Even though none of us would trade the effects of childbirth on our bodies for the precious children we've brought into this world, it doesn't mean that we have to idly accept the ramifications listed above. There *is* something you can do about it! While no suggestions in this book can help shrink the bones of your broadened hips, it *can* help you reduce the amount of fat you store on those hips. This book will also make you a healthier person by changing your eating habits for good, and creating an exercise routine that easily fits into your busy life. You'll also be surprised by the amount of energy you'll have and by the fact that you're not hungry all the time in your effort to lose weight.

In my first book, *Managing Life with Kids*, I discussed some general health issues regarding food and fitness. I quickly realized that this topic needed to be expanded on and deserved a book of its own. There's a lot of confusing information out there and a lot of diet plans that are unnecessarily complicated. Busy moms don't need a diet plan or exercise routine that's difficult to follow. We need a plan that's simple and effective. You'll find this book refreshingly easy to follow and effective to help you reach your weight and fitness goals.

This single book will be all that you need to get on the right track towards attaining your diet goal in just 28 days. It'll teach you what good food choices are to promote weight loss and better health, help you set goals for yourself, educate you with the information you need to lose weight *and* keep it off, create an effective workout program, and provide healthy recipes that will help you maintain your weight goal while providing you and your family with nutritious and delicious meals. The added bonus with this approach to weight loss is that your body will be healthier for it and not deprived of nutrients. You'll also lose weight without starving yourself. That's why this **28 Day Plan** is different from other weight loss programs. This plan works and is easy to maintain for life so you keep off the weight you lose.

I'm not only a Certified Personal Trainer with an additional certification in Pre/Post Natal Training, I'm also a mother of 8 kids who knows time is precious. I've discovered an effective way to lose weight and easily keep it off. I've also created a workout program that will get you in great shape without spending an exorbitant amount of time exercising. I've been involved in fitness practically all my life and have read countless books on general health, diet, exercise, and overall fitness. Even before becoming a trainer myself, I've had personal trainers that I worked with during pregnancy and after childbirth in an attempt to find an effective workout program that allowed me to get maximum results in the limited time I had.

I've had to struggle with my weight all of my life. I definitely was *not* one of those people who could eat whatever she wanted and not gain weight. I've always had to watch what I eat. It used to bother me but then I took on the attitude that it was making me a healthier person. When my friends were eating fast food, I was eating salads. I find it exciting that at my age and with five kids under my belt, I weigh less and look better than I did in high school. (My other three sons I was blessed with through marriage.) What made the difference was getting educated about food and fitness. Growing up I had the discipline but didn't have the information needed to lose weight permanently. We know much more now about weight loss than ever before and using that information to make losing weight easier is the key to success.

I've always had a passion in the area of food and fitness and am excited to provide an all-encompassing book that can help other mothers like you, look and feel their best. You can benefit from all the countless hours of research I've completed and from my own personal experience to help you lose weight and feel great. **Follow the simple plan described in this book and in just 28 days, you'll be leaner, stronger, healthier, and in better shape than ever before!**

CHAPTER 1
CHANGE YOUR MIND, CHANGE YOUR BODY

If you took a poll of 100 people and asked them if they needed to shed some extra pounds, the odds are high that most would say "yes." In fact, it's rare to find someone who is satisfied with their weight. Even with all the money spent in the weight loss industry, people all over the world continue to become overweight. An astonishing two-thirds of Americans are either overweight or obese, making us the fattest country in the world.

You can't pick up a magazine or flip through the channels without being exposed to something regarding weight loss. There are countless exercise products, gyms to join, workout videos, diet pills, and publications geared towards helping people lose weight. So why is it that we're getting fatter each year instead of slimmer? Even our children are gaining weight in epidemic proportions. What's happening?

The simple answer is that we're eating more calories than we're burning but it's more complicated than that. Researchers are trying to determine what has happened in our society today that has created the overweight environment we now live in. Some of what they've discovered is that our society is more sedentary than it used to be, the foods being consumed today have become less healthy and more harmful, the portions of food have increased dramatically, and fewer families are eating meals at home. Put all these factors together and you can't help but to have an overweight society.

WHY LOSING WEIGHT IS IMPORTANT

Being overweight isn't only frustrating from an appearance perspective, it also has serious health ramifications. A society that's overweight is a society that's at high risk for health problems. Listed below are just some of the health risks are that are associated with being overweight or obese:

- **HEART DISEASE**
- **HIGH CHOLESTEROL**
- **ARTHRITIS**
- **GALLSTONES**
- **INFERTILITY**
- **HIGH BLOOD PRESSURE**
- **DIABETES**
- **MOST FORMS OF CANCER**
- **ADULT-ONSET ASTHMA**

The list of health risks continues to grow as researchers discover more about the dangers of being overweight. In fact, your weight is the second most important factor when analyzing your long-term health with smoking being the first to put you at a greater risk for health problems. This statement alone should be enough to motivate anyone to get rid of any extra weight she might be been carrying around.

WHY IT'S SO HARD TO LOSE

There are many factors that contribute to the battle of the bulge. First, as you get older your body needs less calories than it did before and if you don't reduce your caloric intake or add exercise to burn those extra calories, you'll slowly gain weight. We also live in a society that spends hours in front of the TV and computer and pay others to do a lot of our physical labor such as yard work or washing the car. These factors cause us to burn fewer calories just by how we live day-to-day.

It also doesn't help that food portions served at restaurants and the serving sizes of pre-packaged snacks have grown over the years adding unnecessary fat and calories to our diet. Everything now is **SUPERSIZED** and we're encouraged to buy larger portions because it's a better "value." Remember those cute little eight ounce Coke bottles? That was considered a serving size at one time. Now you can get Coke in a 34 ounce bottle. That's over four times the calories. Even though eight ounces should still be considered a single serving, everyone knows that a person is going to drink a lot more if it's served in a larger quantity. You can even purchase a 64 ounce fountain drink at a 7-Eleven called the Double-Gulp. That's eight servings in just one drink and about 750 calories!

Food products have also been **SUPERSIZED**. Candy bars come in king sizes, bags of chips have grown larger and the portion sizes at fast food restaurants have increased dramatically. French fries today are triple what they were in the 1950's and a typical hamburger that used to be one ounce is now six ounces. We're encouraged to eat more just by the nature of the serving size or packaged product. Studies show that the larger the portions of food placed in front of someone, the more he'll eat. This definitely plays a factor in the expansion of America's waist.

Foods also contain more preservatives and other additives the human body doesn't know how to process. Our bodies don't handle processed foods as efficiently as they do natural, or "clean" foods. This means that if your diet consists mostly of foods that contain preservatives and additives, you'll be more likely to gain weight than if you ate clean foods as nature intended. Unfortunately, most of the foods produced today are loaded with all the things our bodies don't need and can't handle which contributes to the fattening of our society.

Food is also associated with fun and prosperity. Everything we do typically involves food – and lots of it! We've all experienced the meal that included far too many options with far too many calories. It's not uncommon for people to leave meals such as Thanksgiving dinner, just as stuffed as the turkey on the table.

An additional obstacle that we mothers face is the fact that when you're raising kids, you're exposed to temptations that you wouldn't normally have *and* you don't always have the time or energy to prepare a healthy meal. As moms, we're tempted by birthday cake far more than most people due to all the birthday parties we attend with our children. Many of us also feel guilty about throwing away the leftover food that our children don't eat and feel the need to finish their plates for them adding extra calories and fat to our diet. We also face the challenge of after attending to all the responsibilities of being a mother, by evening preparing a healthy meal seems daunting and the unhealthy option of fast food does have its appeal.

When you take all this into consideration, it's no wonder that obesity is a major problem today. It's become such a an issue that The World Health Organization announced obesity as a global epidemic having major health implications. Organizations around the world are recognizing that something needs to be done in an effort to stop the increasing weight gain in our society.

Now that we've discussed why we might be carrying around more weight than we should, why it's important to lose that weight, *and* why it's so hard to get the weight off, we can get to the heart of this book which is learning how to lose the weight you want. Whether you want to lose 100 pounds or just that last stubborn five, you'll find out how to overcome the obstacles stated above so you can lose the weight you want *and* keep it off for good. This book is about to make weight loss for you easier than ever before. It's going to do that by first changing your mind about food and exercise which will result in a change in your weight, health and body!

COMMON DIET MYTHS

What we now know about a person's diet, exercise, and weight management is much different than it was ten to twenty years ago. It's undisputable that consuming fewer calories than you burn will assure weight loss, but there are other variables in the equation that can make losing weight easier. If you try to lose weight using outdated information you'll have a harder time shedding pounds versus if you use the information researchers have recently discovered.

Think about all the different diet fads that have made their way around in the last twenty years. There were and still are, countless diets that claim to help you lose weight fast and easy just to have that new "weight loss concept" debunked years later. People at one time avoided all fats and then later were told to eat fats but avoid all carbohydrates. Researchers have discovered that neither is a perfect way to attain weight loss and both come with their own list of health concerns.

Everyone wants the latest secret about how to lose weight easily in hopes that it might help them finally attain their weight goal. When I refer to knowing about the latest research concerning diet and fitness, I'm not talking about some fad diet information. Instead, I'm referring to the scientific research on the balanced intake of healthy foods and having an understanding of how exercise and your metabolism play a role in weight loss and your overall health. Using this up-to-date information and incorporating it into your lifestyle is what's going to help you meet your goals.

To reach your weight loss goals you also have to change how you view food and exercise. If you do this, losing weight and eating healthy will be easier than you ever thought. For example, some people think of exercise as something they *have* to do in order to lose weight. Rather, it should be seen as an activity that's invigorating and makes you feel great while at the same time strengthens your body and also aids in weight loss. On the same note regarding food, watermelon should be viewed as an equal dessert to a double fudge chocolate cake. You might not think that now but by the time you complete my *Clean and Lean in 28 Days™* plan, you will. You'll see how nature's candy, such as watermelon and other sweet fruits, are just as satisfying as a fat-filled dessert which can leave you stuffed and guilt-ridden after eating it. You'll start to think of food as fuel to help your body become healthy and strong and start eating only to satisfy hunger and not to become satiated. *Lose Weight, Feel Great!* is going to change your mind which will result in a beautiful change in your body.

We'll start now by cleansing your brain of the following common diet myths:

1. FACT OR FICTION?
Eat three square meals a day.
Fiction. It's now known that eating three small meals a day with a snack in between is a better way to fuel your body and increase your metabolism. (Your metabolism is an important factor in losing weight and will be discussed at length later in the book.) By eating three small meals and two snacks every day, you'll have better success at losing weight because not only will your metabolism continue to burn calories at a steady rate, but you won't feel excessively hungry since you get to eat something every three to four hours. This prevents binge eating and helps you stay on track. "Snacking" can have bad connotations but the snacks you eat need to be healthy and should contain approximately 150 calories each. (In *Chapter 4 - Three Successful Keys to Weight-Loss*, we'll discuss in detail how to properly incorporate snacks into your diet plan.)

2. FACT OR FICTION?
Eating a large dinner is a normal part of a healthy diet.
Fiction. This is the exact opposite of what is true. Dinner should be the *smallest* meal of the day and breakfast should be the largest. Follow the adage, "Eat breakfast like a king, lunch like a prince, and dinner like a pauper." Your body's metabolism peaks around 12:00 p.m. and then slows down as the day progresses. With that in mind, it only makes sense to consume most of your calories early and then reduce your caloric intake later in the day. If you eat a large meal for supper, your body will store what it doesn't need which will hurt your weight loss effort and contribute to weight gain. It's better to eat a large breakfast to jump start your metabolism, have a reasonably sized lunch, and then eat just a small meal for supper.

3. FACT OR FICTION?
Avoid all fats.
Fiction. You need fat! It plays a vital part in how your body operates from supplying the building blocks for hormones that control all of your body's life processes, to transporting fat-soluble vitamins and phytochemicals from your intestines to your bloodstream. Fats are also great for healthy hair and are essential in maintaining good health. Fats fall either under the label of a good fat or a bad fat. Your body doesn't need bad fats, but it must have the good fats to operate. Good fats can be found in food sources such as olive oil, avocadoes, walnuts,

almonds, and salmon. Consuming good fats improves your health and can reduce the risk of heart disease. In regards to losing weight, good fats don't raise your insulin levels which is important for weight loss and overall health. They're also great at suppressing your appetite and slowing down the digestive process which helps keep you feeling fuller longer. (The good fats and bad fats will be discussed further in the next chapter.)

4. FACT OR FICTION?
Avoid all carbohydrates.

Fiction. This is a myth that's out there as a result of the Atkins Diet. This diet plan had people eating all the bacon they wanted yet discouraged eating healthy fruits and vegetables. Like fats, there are good carbs and there are bad carbs. You want to avoid the bad carbs which consist of white products such as white pasta, white rice, white potatoes, white bread, white flour, and any white flour products. Pure sugar is at the top of the bad carb list. White carbs, or simple carbohydrates, are highly refined and have been linked to weight gain, heart disease, type 2 diabetes, and many cancers due to the speed in which they're digested and enter your bloodstream as sugar. This process has a very negative effect on your body's metabolism.

On the other hand, good carbs contain plenty of fiber, vitamins, minerals, and phytochemicals to fight diseases and promote overall good health. Good carbs consist of whole grains such as brown rice, 100% whole wheat bread, whole wheat pasta, beans, fruits, and non-starchy vegetables. These carbs are digested slowly releasing insulin in a regulated manner. The slower a food is digested, the better it is for your body. Good carbs help reduce the risk of heart disease, lower your risk of cancer, protect against type 2 diabetes, improve your gastrointestinal health, and aid in weight loss. This is why cutting all carbs out of your diet isn't a good idea. You just have to eat the right ones. *(A list of good carbs can be found in Chapter 2 – What to Eat and What to Avoid.)*

5. FACT OR FICTION?
Eat dairy products when trying to lose weight.

Fact. People used to avoid dairy products when trying to lose weight but recent studies claim that dairy products actually help to *promote* weight loss. A recent study showed that obese adults who ate a high-dairy diet lost more weight and fat than those who ate a low-dairy diet even though both groups consumed the same amount of calories. The study claims that eating three to four servings of dairy a day increases the fat breakdown in cells and promotes weight loss. The dairy products need to be low-fat, if not fat-free, to be effective. This study is still under dispute but regardless of the findings, you should still make healthy dairy products such as low-fat yogurt, low-fat cottage cheese, and skim milk, an important part of your diet because they provide some of the vitamins and nutrients your body needs.

6. FACT OR FICTION?
All low-fat and fat-free products are great options for dieters.

Fiction. This is a common misconception that many people have. Even though we stated above that low-fat and fat-free dairy products are good, that's not the case for many other foods.

Many of the "fat-free" processed and packaged foods will have the same amount of calories if not *more* calories than their counterparts that contain more fat. Also, many dieters feel as if they have the green light to eat more since they know it's low-fat, and ultimately consume more calories. You need to carefully read the labels of foods that claim to be low-fat or fat-free to determine if it's a good food option because many times, it's not.

7. FACT OR FICTION?

Salad bars are always a good option for a low calorie meal.

Fiction. For a diet-friendly salad, stay clear of fattening dressings, pasta and macaroni salads, fried croutons, nuts, and cheeses because they are so high in fat and calories. In fact, the average woman consumes most of her fat intake in the form of salad dressings, not French fries or other greasy foods like you might think. A salad can end of being just as fattening as a burger and fries if you're not careful. To reap the benefits of all the wonderful nutrients like lycopene and beta-carotene that are found in salads you need a *little* fat to help your body absorb them. Olive oil and vinegar, low fat dressing, low fat cheeses, a few nuts, or boiled eggs are all healthy options. Be careful however, not to overdo it.

8. FACT OR FICTION?

Nuts are too high in fat and calories to be part of a weight loss program.

Fiction. This used to be the thought process of every dieter out there. Now we know better. Yes, nuts have a lot of fat but it's the kind of fat your body thrives on protecting it from countless ailments and diseases. Nuts are also great at keeping hunger at bay because they are high in protein. When eaten in moderation, nuts can play an important role in your weight loss goal. I personally have experienced the wonderful effects of this nutrient powerhouse. I used to be scared to eat nuts but now knowing the latest information, I've eaten more in the past two years than I had over the past fifteen. I've also experienced more weight loss success than ever before. That's proof enough for me! In fact, I always keep a can of low-salt mixed nuts in my car to snack on while I'm running around picking up kids here and there. Having a healthy snack prevents my hunger from tempting me to succumb to all the junk that's out there or binge eating when I get home.

9. FACT OR FICTION?

In order to lose weight, you have to stay hungry all the time.

Fiction. If you find yourself always hungry on any type of diet, odds are very high that even if you lose weight, you'll quickly regain it. Our bodies are meant to respond to hunger pangs and unless you are incredibly disciplined, you'll yield to the cries of your body and eat. Many times people that have starved themselves end up binge eating and consume far too many calories in one sitting.

It's much more effective and long lasting to respond to your hunger in a modest way. This concept goes back to the point made earlier about eating three small meals a day along with two snacks. If you eat five times throughout the day, your body gets the fuel it needs and you'll stay fuller longer. The only time you should ever resist the real urge to give into hunger pangs is late at night. If you do feel hungry after your last meal, try drinking a lot of water which can help eliminate your cravings. Other than resisting the urge to eat late at night, you shouldn't feel intense hunger even when trying to lose weight.

Hopefully, this clears up some the misconceptions about food and diet to get you in the right frame of mind towards weight loss. It's important to understand some of the fundamentals of food and nutrition to maximize the effort you put into your weight loss program. As busy mothers, we know we need the most effective game plan to get into shape because our time and energy is limited. We want maximum results with minimal effort and knowing the facts can help us accomplish our goal.

CHAPTER 2
FOODS FOR SUCCESSFUL DIETING
WHAT TO EAT & WHAT TO AVOID

Calorie for calorie, all foods are not created equal. As discussed in the previous chapter, a bowl of white pasta affects our bodies negatively, whereas a bowl of wheat pasta does not. Even though they contain the same amount of calories, the wheat pasta is better for your body and can be an important part of your weight loss effort. It's not always just about the *quantity* of what we eat but also the *quality*.

WHAT DETERMINES THE QUALITY OF A CERTAIN FOOD?

1. GLYCEMIC INDEX. The term glycemic index (GI) is becoming more and more popular. Some products now even list it on their packaging due to the rise in consumer awareness. A food's glycemic index is one of the major factors that determine the impact a food has on your body. A food's GI is a measure of how various foods affect your blood sugar level. If a food is high on the GI chart, it's quickly digested. This means that the food is rapidly converted into sugar which is NOT what you want to have happen. If a food has a low GI number, it's slowly digested which is better on your metabolic system and helpful in your weight loss attempt because it allows you to feel fuller longer. GI is measured on a scale from 0-100. Pure sugar is the highest with a GI of 100 and tomatoes are near the bottom of the scale with a GI of only 15. The lower the GI the better a food is for your body.

2. ENERGY DENSITY. Another factor to consider when determining a food's impact on your body's health is the food's energy density. If a food has a high energy density, it means that it contains a large number of calories in a small volume. For example, candies, desserts, and processed foods have very high energy density while fruits and vegetables have a very low energy density level. The more foods you consume with low energy density, the more weight you'll lose because you'll be satisfied with fewer calories. You can eat a larger amount of low density foods while consuming fewer calories than if you consumed the same amount of high density foods. That's because high density foods are more concentrated in calories. The two factors that help a food contain fewer calories while also being more filling are (1) the amount of water it contains and (2) the amount of fiber it provides. Water provides volume but not calories. Grapefruit is 90% water and only has about 40 calories per serving size. One cup of carrots is only around 50 calories and is made up of 88% water. The amount of fiber found in a food is also important. High fiber foods such as whole grains, fruits, and vegetables provide volume and take longer to digest making you feel fuller longer. Please note how many times the phrase "feeling fuller longer" has already been mentioned in this book. That's because it's a major key in your weight loss success. The fuller you are, the less you'll consume. This is why it's so important to educate yourself about which foods can help you accomplish your weight loss goal and then to make those foods a major part of your diet.

3. PROCESS LEVEL. The more processed a food is, the less nutritional value it contains and the harder it is for your body to digest. Your body can maximize the value of natural foods more efficiently than ones containing artificial additives and preservatives. Therefore, you always want to choose foods that are free of artificial ingredients. The excessive amount of processed food that's consumed in our society is becoming more and more of a problem and is contributing to the rise of the obesity level and other health issues. Researchers continue to find a correlation between unhealthy eating and diseases . For this reason, it's imperative that you make good food choices for you *and* your family to maintain a healthy body. Life is much different now than it was for our grandparents who ate straight from the farm with fresh milk, meat, and vegetables. Companies have created artificial additives and preservatives in order to prolong shelf life and supposedly improve a food's taste and make for better packaging and shipping of products. Growth hormones and antibiotics are also widely used to create bigger profits for companies yet they create even more health concerns for our society. The chemicals, preservatives, and additives we're consuming all have an adverse effect on our health and our weight. Reducing, if not completely eliminating processed foods from your diet, will aid in weight loss and greatly improve your overall health.

HOW TO CHOOSE HEALTHY FOODS:

• **ELIMINATE FOODS WITH PARTIALLY HYDROGENATED OILS.** Partially hydrogenated oils are a form of trans fats. Trans fats have been linked to type 2 diabetes, cardiovascular disease, breast cancer, infertility and other health ailments. When purchasing any food product you should closely inspect the ingredients. Just because the package says "0 trans fats" it doesn't mean that the product is safe. The FDA allows for food manufacturers to claim that their products are "trans fat free" if there is less than 0.5 grams of trans fat per serving. A product might make this claim and yet still contain partially hydrogenated oils. The problem here is first researchers are still unclear if *any* consumption is safe. The FDA has told us to consume *no more* than two grams per day but this number is still under scrutiny. Secondly, the serving sizes are so small that people rarely consume just one serving. If a serving has .4 grams of trans fats and you consume two servings in a sitting, you've taken in almost half of what the FDA *thinks* might be safe. Also, if you consume a little trans fat here and there, by the end of the day you can easily exceed the recommended maximum in take of two grams. Therefore, even if the packaging claims to have "zero trans fats", read the ingredient label to see if the product contains partially hydrogenated oil. If it does, avoid it. Eliminating this evil fat will not only help you attain your weight goal, but also improve your overall health.

• **AVOID FOOD PRESERVATIVES SUCH AS BHA, BHT, TBHQ, AND SODIUM NITRATE.** These preservatives are commonly found in cereals, most processed foods, and luncheon meats. Read food labels for these ingredients and avoid them as much as possible. Some of the health issues these preservatives have been linked to include an increase in the risks of cancer, negative effects on liver and kidney function, an increase in blood cholesterol levels, birth defects in lab rats, tumors, and hyperactivity. In fact, because of the associated health risks BHA, BHT, and TBHQ they have been *banned* in some countries.

• **AVOID HIGH FRUCTOSE CORN SYRUP.** This ingredient has not only been linked to an increase in the risk of diabetes, but also triggers your brain into thinking you're still hungry even if you're not. This fact alone can lead to overeating and obesity since you need your brain to signal you to stop eating. Studies have also shown that high fructose corn syrup can raise triglyceride levels in your bloodstream which can increase the risk of heart disease. This ingredient is found in a wide range of products including juice boxes, sports drinks, yogurts and salad dressings. Once you start reading ingredient labels you'll be shocked to find how many products contain high fructose corn syrup. It's difficult to *completely* avoid it, but you can at least choose the products that don't list it as one of the first few ingredients. The ingredients of a product are listed in descending order of predominance by weight. This means that choosing a food with high fructose corn syrup listed at the end of the ingredient list is a much better choice than one that has it as the first ingredient.

• **AVOID WHITE PRODUCTS.** Buy only grain products that have the words "whole" or "bran" mentioned in the list of ingredients. Other grains are considered refined and offer very little nutritional value and will hamper your weight loss effort. As mentioned earlier, white products such as white bread, white pasta, white rice, white flour and white sugar, quickly enter your bloodstream as sugar and adversely affect your metabolism. White products are highly refined and are associated with weight gain, heart disease, type 2 diabetes and many cancers. The healthy and diet friendly grains of choice are whole wheat bread, wheat pastas, wheat flour products, and brown rice.

• **LIMIT YOUR INTAKE OF ARTIFICIAL SWEETENERS.** Many people view artificial sweeteners as a dieter's dream but the verdict is still out on their safety and effectiveness on weight loss. Each type of artificial sweetener comes with its own health concerns and some studies have shown that there's an actual *increase* in appetite when zero calorie sweeteners are consumed. Another negative is that most artificial sweeteners are up to 700 times sweeter than table sugar. Consuming this high concentration of sweetness can distort our natural taste for the sweetness of foods. When your taste buds are used to eating foods and beverages with artificial sweeteners, naturally sweet foods such as oranges and blueberries, will lose their appeal because their taste will pale in comparison to the elevated sweetness you're used to. If you need to sweeten your foods or beverages, you're better off using real sugar and trying to limit the amount. For example, if you like sugar in your tea, try to gradually decrease the amount you use over time in an effort to cut calories. If you *must* use an artificial sweetener, so far sucralose (Splenda) seems to be the lesser of the evils because it's derived from real sugar and is fully absorbed into your system unlike other sweeteners. Two other good choices are stevia and truvia which are non-caloric, and are derived from natural herbs that are used as a sweetener. They can typically be found at health food stores and high-end grocery stores.

• **CHOOSE YOUR CEREAL WISELY.** The cereal aisle is probably the most challenging aisle to shop when it comes to selecting a healthy product. Even the cereals that claim to promote good health and would seem to be a wise choice, can contain partially hydrogenated oils and preservatives. The preservative BHT is added to almost all mainstream cereals so carefully check the ingredients.

(You'll typically find it on the last line of a cereal's nutritional information guide.) The best choices for cereals are found in health foods stores or on the health food aisle at your local grocer. You will find a few mainstream cereals that are free of additives and preservatives labeled "organic" or a few on the top of the cereal aisle. Due to increased consumer awareness, more and more healthy options are becoming available. Carefully read the labels on the cereal boxes to determine which are safe to consume. Choose the cereals that are high in fiber and protein and low in sugar to help aid in your weight loss effort. Be cautious of the caloric and fat content of some of the "health food" cereals. They're good for you but can pack a lot of fat and calories. When I chose these cereals, I cut my serving size in half to compensate for their high calorie and fat content.

• **SHOP THE PERIMETER OF GROCERY STORES.** Shopping the perimeter of a store is an easy way to keep things healthy. This is where you'll find fruits, vegetables, dairy, fish, meats, and breads. These are for the most part, natural foods and not of the processed variety. Once you have figured out what the good food choices are, your shopping actually becomes easier because many of the items in the store are no longer an option.

• **BEWARE OF THE BEVERAGES YOU DRINK.** Beverages should be scrutinized the same way you would your food choices. The large amount of beverage options available now is amazing. There are many drinks to choose from so you have to be aware of which ones will do your body good and which ones will just fill you up with empty calories. Again, reading labels is the best way to determine exactly what's going into your body. If a drink contains a lot of calories or harmful ingredients with no nutritional value, you're better off drinking something else - preferably water.

LIMIT, IF NOT ELIMINATE, YOUR INTAKE OF SOFT DRINKS.

Soft drinks offer no nutritional benefit. In fact, studies have shown that they may actually be detrimental to a person's health. This holds true for the regular soft drinks as well as the low-calorie ones. Just because it's a diet soda doesn't mean it's an acceptable beverage choice for your weight loss effort or overall health. As discussed in the section on artificial sweeteners, a diet soft drink's artificial sweetness can actually cause you to develop a taste for overly sweet foods. They may also increase your appetite. If your family consumes these chemical-laden drinks on a regular basis, you should try to reduce your consumption of them as much as possible. An occasional soft drink here and there is fine, but don't buy soft drinks to be consumed regularly in your home.

LIMIT SPORTS DRINK CONSUMPTION.

In the media we constantly hear about how sedentary our youth has become and that child obesity is becoming an epidemic, yet sports drinks now constitute a larger portion of beverage sales than ever before and are commonly consumed by our youth. These beverages were originally created as a drink to be consumed after or while engaging in strenuous activity. Today's children are drinking sports drinks on a regular basis regardless of their activity level. They're hurting themselves in two areas because not only are they consuming the unnecessary extra calories from sports drinks, they're also missing out on other beverages that are good for them. This holds true for adults as well.

LIMIT YOUR ALCOHOL CONSUMPTION.

If you choose to consume alcohol your best choice is red wine, followed by white wine then light beer. Keep your consumption to a minimum because alcohol adds extra calories, dehydrates your body, and can weaken your discipline causing you to make poor food choices and overeat.

DRINK PLENTY OF WATER.

Water should make up the majority of your liquid intake. The benefits of water are amazing and range from helping you lose weight, to achieving great skin and hair. Water is necessary for your body to operate and thrive properly. It aids in your body's metabolism and also helps you feel full. In fact, sometimes the hunger pangs you feel are caused by a water deficiency or dehydration and can be satisfied with water. When you feel a sense of hunger, drink 8-16 ounces of water, wait 20 minutes and then determine if you are still truly hungry. To get the maximum benefits of water you should drink at least eight, 8 ounce glasses a day.

I might have mentioned some additives and preservatives that you never considered a health hazard, but you should really consider the role they play in your diet. Many people think that since these artificial ingredients are commonly found in foods, they must be safe to consume. This could not be further from the truth. A perfect example of why it's important to educate yourself about what's in the foods you eat is the recent attention to trans fats. Approximately 11 years prior to the FDA mandating that food manufacturers list the amount of trans fats on their nutritional information label, certain groups had researched their associated risks. The recommendation of the research was to avoid the consumption of *all* partially hydrogenated oils. It took the FDA over 11 years from when I'd first read about trans fat for them to address the dangerous health issues linked to this ingredient so commonly found in foods. Fortunately for my family, I was aware of the research conducted and avoided consuming this dangerous fat for over a decade before it was addressed by the FDA. This is why educating yourself about what you eat and drink and not relying on food companies or government agencies for information is the best defense in an effort to keep you and your family healthy and maintain a healthy weight.

In the following charts, you'll find listed for each food group the best options to maximize your weight loss effort as well as to promote better health. The foods found in the "worst" column should be completely avoided if possible. If that isn't realistic for you, then the amount consumed should be kept to a minimum. Keep in mind that the closer you follow the plan in this book, the sooner you'll reach the results you want. *(Please note that I always recommend buying organic products whenever possible. It's more nutritious, and free of hormones and pesticides.)*

DAIRY PRODUCTS

BEST	WORST
Skim milk	Whole milk
1% milk	Full-fat cheeses
Soy milk *(plain)*	Cream
Almond milk	Ice cream
Yogurt *(low-fat)* *plain has less sugar	Butter
Part-skim mozzarella cheese	Margarine
Low-fat cottage cheese	
Parmesan cheese	
Eggs *(Omega -3 fortified are the best. My favorite is **Eggland's Best**)*	
Low-fat frozen yogurt	
Smart Balance Plus Butter Spread *(when butter is needed)*	

PROTEINS

BEST	WORST
Walnuts	Fried chicken, or seafood
Almonds	Fatty cuts of beef or pork
Brazil nuts	Ground beef
Pine nuts	Hot dogs
Cashews	Sausage
Soy nuts	Bacon
Other nuts and seeds	Processed meats *(this includes deli meats)*
Fish	
Shellfish	
Skinless chicken	
Extra-lean or lean ground turkey breast or ground beef	
Lean cuts of beef *(filets, flank steak, top round, London broil)*	
Tofu	
Soy dogs	

CARBOHYDRATES

BEST	WORST
100% whole wheat bread *(Be aware of wheat breads that don't have 100% or "whole" in front of it because it's just about the same as refined flour and should be avoided.)* Brown rice Whole wheat pasta Whole wheat couscous Whole grain cereal Oatmeal Beans Lentils Peas	White bread White rice White pasta Plain bagels Biscuits Pretzels and chips White flour products White pizza dough Sugary cereals Doughnuts and other desserts

VEGETABLES

PREFERRED	LIMIT
Broccoli Brussels sprouts Cabbage Collards Cauliflower Asparagus Spinach Romaine lettuce Arugula Red lettuce and other darker lettuces Tomatoes Bell peppers Red and yellow onions Green beans Yellow squash Zucchini	White potatoes Corn

FRUITS

PREFERRED	LIMIT
Blueberries	Bananas
Strawberries	Pineapples
Raspberries	Mangos
Pears	Papayas
Cantaloupe	Fruit juices *(these have a concentrated level of sugar with high caloric content)*
Cherries	
Apples	Dried fruit *(same as juices)*
Grapefruit	Canned or frozen fruit with added sugar or syrup
Oranges	
Tangerines	
Plums	
Cherries	
Red grapes	

BEVERAGES

BEST	WORST
Water	All soft drinks *(this includes diet)*
Skim milk	Sugar-fortified sports drinks
Green tea	Fruit juices
Black tea	Commercial fruit smoothies
Coffee *(without sugar)*	Full calorie beers
100% vegetable juices *(reduced-sodium)*	Sugary alcoholic drinks
Red wine	
Light beers *(if you must)*	

CHAPTER 3
KNOWING YOUR NUMBERS

Losing weight is all about numbers; it's a simple mathematical equation. To lose weight, you must consume fewer calories than you burn. If you take in more calories than your body needs, you'll gain weight. It's really not that complicated.

With the simple formulas in this chapter, you'll find it easy to calculate what you need to do to lose weight. This chapter will focus on helping you determine exactly how many calories you need to restrict yourself to in order to lose the weight you want. You'll calculate how many calories you need to cut from your daily consumption and how much exercise you need to add to hit your 28 day goal. There are seven easy steps in this chapter to help you figure out exactly what you need to do to start losing weight today. These steps include:

1. Calculating your **BMR** (basal metabolic rate)
2. Calculating your total caloric needs based on your current weight.
3. Calculating your **BMI** (body mass index).
4. Determining your frame size.
5. Setting a weight goal.
6. Calculating the daily calories allowed to reach your weight goal.
7. Calculating how many calories you're allowed to maintain your goal weight.

Calculating what your caloric needs should be makes weight loss easier because you know exactly what your food consumption is supposed to be. Following these steps for weight loss is like taking a long car trip. When you decide to go somewhere, just because you know what your destination is, or in this case what your weight goal is, it doesn't mean you'll get there. You need a map and directions to get you where you want to go. For weight loss, just knowing your goal won't get you there either. You have to know the numbers that are involved to reach your goal. If you're not a "numbers person", don't be intimidated by these formulas because they're simple to follow and critical in setting you up for weight loss success.

You'll find the 7 steps listed below to help you determine what your numbers are, what you need to do to achieve your goal weight, and how to keep the weight off. At the end of this chapter you'll find a chart you can use to input the numbers you've calculated for easy reference.

STEP 1: CALCULATING YOUR BASAL METABOLIC RATE

First, you need to determine your basal metabolic rate, or **BMR**. This number represents the amount of calories your body needs just to stay alive. Put another way, it's the amount of calories your body needs for the functioning of vital organs while at rest. This number declines as you age due to natural muscle mass loss and the aging process itself. Your **BMR** will also decline as you lose weight because your body has less weight to carry around on a daily basis and needs fewer calories to exist. This said, you need to recalculate your **BMR** as you lose weight and as you age. To determine what your number is, use the formula below:

HARRIS BENEDICT ENGLISH BMR FORMULA

Women: **BMR** = 655 + (4.35 x wt. in pounds) + (4.7 x ht. in inches) − (4.7 x age in years)

Men: **BMR** = 66 + (6.23 x wt. in pounds) + (12.7 x ht. in inches) − (6.8 x age in years)

STEP 2: CALCULATING YOUR TOTAL DAILY CALORIC NEEDS

Second, take your **BMR**, and put into the equation how many more calories your body needs as a result of your physical activity. This will give you your **Adjusted BMR**, or your total daily caloric needs. Be honest with yourself and calculate how much exercise you actually participate in and not how much exercise you *hope* you'll accomplish. The number you come up with is the amount of calories you need to maintain your *current* weight. This number will be used later to help you determine how many calories you need to limit yourself to in order to achieve your weight goal.

AMOUNT OF EXERCISE	CALCULATE =
Little or no exercise	**BMR** x 1.2
Light exercise *(1-3 days a week)*	**BMR** x 1.375
Moderate exercise *(3-5 days a week)*	**BMR** x 1.55
Hard exercise *(6-7 days a week)*	**BMR** x 1.725
Very hard exercise *(very hard exercise, a physical job or training twice a day)*	**BMR** x 1.9

STEP 3: CALCULATING YOUR BODY MASS INDEX

Your body mass index, or **BMI**, is calculated by using your weight and height. **BMI** is a relatively reliable indicator of a healthy body weight for an individual. Most physicians prefer to use **BMI** to estimate the weight category of their patients. **BMI** is broken down into five different categories to determine whether a person is underweight, healthy, overweight, obese or morbidly obese. Like most formulas, **BMI** also has its limitations. It has a range of error that can be effected by a person's advanced age, very young age, and a person with a very high percentage of muscle mass. Even with its limitations, **BMI** is still the perferred method of establishing a person's ideal weight. Again, these formulas are to be used as a guide. Common sense and your mirror are your best measuring tools.

CALCULATING YOUR BMI:

1. Multiply your weight in pounds by x 703
2. Divide this number by your height in inches
3. Divide the number again by your height in inches to get your **BMI**

An example of this formula for a women who's 5 foot 5 inches and weighs 125 pounds would be (125 x 703) divided by 65 = 1,352. Then 1,352 divided by 65 = 20.8. By using the chart below, you see that her **BMI** puts her in the healthy category without being borderline over or underweight.

Take your calculated **BMI** and use the chart to find the category in which your number falls. Determine if you're in the middle of the range for the given category, the bottom or the top to get an even better picture of where you stand.

BMI CATEGORIES:

below 18.5	underweight
18.5 - 24.9	healthy
25.0 - 29.9	overweight
30.0 - 39.9	obese
over 40	morbidly obese

STEP 4: DETERMINING YOUR FRAME SIZE

The following method is used by Metropolitan Life Insurance Company to calculate frame size.

1. Bend your arm at a 90° angle in front of your body with forearm parallel to the floor.

2. Keep your fingers straight and turn the inside of your wrist towards your body.

3. Place your thumb and index finger on the two prominent bones on either side of your elbow, then measure the distance between the bones with a tape measure.

4. Compare your number to the chart below which states the measurement for a medium frame. If your elbow measurement for your particular height is less than the number of inches listed, you have a small frame. If your elbow measurement is more than the number of inches, you have a large frame.

ELBOW MEASUREMENT: FOR MEDIUM FRAMES

WOMEN HEIGHT	ELBOW MEASUREMENT	MEN HEIGHT	ELBOW MEASUREMENT
4' 10" – 4' 11"	2-1/4" to 2-1/2"	5' 2" – 5' 3"	2-1/2" to 2-7/8"
5' 0" – 5' 3"	2-1/4" to 2-1/2"	5' 4" – 5' 7"	2-5/8" to 2-7/8"
5' 4" – 5' 7"	2-3/8" to 2-5/8"	5' 8" – 5' 11"	2-3/4" to 3"
5' 8" – 5' 11"	2-3/8" to 2-5/8"	6' 0" – 6' 3"	2-3/4" to 3-1/8"
6' 0"	2-1/2" to 2-3/4"	6' 4"	2-7/8" to 3-1/4"

STEP 5: SETTING A WEIGHT GOAL

There's no hard and fast rule as to exactly what a person should weigh. There are many factors that have to be taken into consideration. No matter what the charts below state as the "ideal" weight range for a given height, the mirror is your best indicator. Don't get trapped into the mindset of locking in on a specific number and lose focus on the fact that you're trying to get healthy, feel good, and look your best. Use good judgement and common sense when trying to attain a weight that's best for you. Also keep in mind that muscle is heavier by volume than fat. As you develop more muscle mass by following this book's workout program, don't get frustrated if at first the scale doesn't drop like you want it. Let the mirror be your guide. Initially, you might weigh a pound or two more than when you started, but actually appear to have lost weight since having toned muscles is slenderizing.

With that said, the charts below will give you a general idea of a target weight. I have listed two "ideal weight" charts. The first was put out by Met Life in 1983. It uses your frame size, height and gender to give you a weight range. I personally feel that the charts error by being more forgiving of extra weight on women, and less forgiving on men. I almost left out the Met Life charts because I do feel they have a certain degree of error but they're so commonly referred to, I felt I needed to include them. The second set of charts is more current and was developed by *The University of Wisconsin Medical School*. **Use the charts to help set a weight goal for you.**

WEIGHT CHART FOR WOMEN
Weight in pounds, based on ages 25 - 59 with the lowest mortality rate
(indoor clothing weighing 3 pounds and shoes with 1" heels)

Height	Small Frame	Medium Frame	Large Frame
4'10"	102 - 111	109 - 121	118 - 131
4'11"	103 - 113	111 - 123	120 - 134
5'0"	104 - 115	113 - 126	122 - 137
5'1"	106 - 118	115 - 129	125 - 140
5'2"	108 - 121	118 - 132	128 - 143
5'3"	111 - 124	121 - 135	131 - 147
5'4"	114 - 127	124 - 138	134 - 151
5'5"	117 - 130	127 - 141	137 - 155
5'6"	120 - 133	130 - 144	140 - 159
5'7"	123 - 136	133 - 147	143 - 163
5'8"	126 - 139	136 - 150	146 - 167
5'9"	129 - 142	139 - 153	149 - 170
5'10"	132 - 145	142 - 156	152 - 173
5'11"	135 - 148	145 - 159	155 - 176
6'0"	138 - 151	148 - 162	158 - 179

WEIGHT CHART FOR MEN
Weight in pounds, based on ages 25 - 59 with the lowest mortality rate
(indoor clothing weighing 5 pounds and shoes with 1" heels)

Height	Small Frame	Medium Frame	Large Frame
5'2"	128 - 134	131 - 141	138 - 150
5'3"	130 - 136	133 - 143	140 - 153
5'4"	132 - 138	135 - 145	142 - 156
5'5"	134 - 140	137 - 148	144 - 160
5'6"	136 - 142	139 - 151	146 - 164
5'7"	138 - 145	142 - 154	149 - 168
5'8"	140 - 148	145 - 157	152 - 172
5'9"	142 - 151	148 - 160	155 - 176
5'10"	144 - 154	151 - 163	158 - 180
5'11"	146 - 157	154 - 166	161 - 184
6'0"	149 - 160	157 - 170	164 - 188
6'1"	152 - 164	160 - 174	168 - 192
6'2"	155 - 168	164 - 178	172 - 197
6'3"	158 - 172	167 - 182	176 - 202
6'4"	162 - 176	171 - 187	181 - 207

IDEAL WEIGHT FOR MEN AND WOMEN:
BASED ON BODY MASS INDEX
(The University of Wisconsin Medical School)

According to physicians, a person's ideal weight would fall inside the healthy weight range for women and men as defined by the **Body Mass Index (BMI)**. This healthy range is between 18.5 and 24.9. If you're a woman, you should look at the lower numbers of the ideal range just as a man should determine his ideal weight from the higher numbers.

BODY MASS INDEX

Height (ft/inches)	Ideal Weight (Pounds)
5' 0"	97 - 127
5' 1"	100 - 132
5' 2"	103 - 136
5' 3"	107 - 140
5' 4"	110 - 145
5' 5"	113 - 149
5' 6"	117 - 154
5' 7"	121 - 159
5' 8"	124 - 164
5' 9"	128 - 168
5' 10"	132 - 173
5' 11"	135 - 178
6' 0"	139 - 183

The following charts give a specific ideal weight for each gender based on a healthy body-fat percentage for women and men.

IDEAL WEIGHT FOR WOMEN BASED ON BODY-FAT PERCENT	
Height (ft/inches)	**Ideal Weight** (Pounds)
5' 0"	100
5' 1"	105
5' 2"	110
5' 3"	115
5' 4"	120
5' 5"	125
5' 6"	130
5' 7"	135
5' 8"	140
5' 9"	145
5' 10"	150
5' 11"	155
6' 0"	160

IDEAL WEIGHT FOR MEN BASED ON BODY-FAT PERCENTAGE	
Height (ft/inches)	**Ideal Weight** (Pounds)
5' 0"	106
5' 1"	112
5' 2"	118
5' 3"	124
5' 4"	130
5' 5"	136
5' 6"	142
5' 7"	148
5' 8"	154
5' 9"	160
5' 10"	166
5' 11"	172
6' 0"	178
6' 1"	184
6' 2"	190
6' 3"	196
6' 4"	202

STEP 6: CALCULATING THE DAILY CALORIES ALLOWED TO REACH YOUR WEIGHT GOAL

This is one of the most important steps in knowing your numbers and having weight loss success. In this step, you'll determine exactly how many calories you need to restrict yourself to in order to lose the weight you want in 28 days. You'll also be able to establish your daily caloric needs to reach your *long* term weight loss goal.

In order to reach your goal, you need to follow the steps in the chart below to determine the amount of calories you need to cut based on how many pounds you want to lose. Remember that a pound equals 3,500 calories. Therefore, if you cut back 500 calories a day you'll lose one pound per week. You can use the chart below to determine your caloric intake or to reach your goal faster, you can cut back to 1200 calories per day. NEVER go below 1200 calories. If your **BMR** is extremely high, this number may be too low for you initially, so adjust it to a reasonable goal. You want to reach your weight goal over a realistic amount of time and keep the weight off for good. If cutting back to 1200 calories per day is too severe, try 1500 calories. It's important to stick with your diet plan and you're more likely to do so if it's realistic. However, if you're motivated and ready to shed that extra weight faster, 1200 calories is a great way to do it. **(Remember to consult your physician before starting any weight-loss program.)**

In the chart below, record all the numbers you've calculated so far regarding your weight and goals. Use this information to determine the amount of calories that you're allowed to meet your new weight goal. If the number you get for your total calories is below 1200, your goal is unrealistic. Adjust the number to 1200 and understand that it will take time to lose all the weight you want but you will be losing at a healthy pace and will be more likely to keep it off.

KNOWING YOUR NUMBERS CHART:

Current weight	
Current adjusted **BMR**	
Frame size	
28 day Weight goal	
Pounds to lose in 28 days	
(Pounds to lose x 3,500) divided by 28 days = *This is how many calories you need to cut each day to attain your 28 day goal. You can do this by reducing your daily caloric intake and increasing how much you exercise.	
Caloric goal per day (Subtract the above number from your current adjusted **BMR** to determine how many calories you should be restricted to each day.)	

To further your effort in weight loss, adding physical activity is paramount. You can double your effort by cutting calories and exercising to burn off even more calories. If you cut back 500 calories a day and exercise enough to burn an extra 500 calories, you'll double your weight loss and lose two pounds per week instead of one. Adding exercise to your diet program will also increase your **BMR** helping you to burn more calories even when you're not exercising. Remember when you lose weight *and* as you get older, your **BMR** declines so it's always good to recalculate your numbers and add exercise or cut your caloric intake to adjust for the reduction in your **BMR**. This will help ensure that you don't gradually let extra pounds creep up on you over the years. *(Chapter 7 – Creating a Workout Program, will discuss how to incorporate exercise into your weight loss goals in more detail.)*

STEP 7: CALCULATING HOW MANY CALORIES YOU'RE ALLOWED TO MAINTAIN YOUR WEIGHT GOAL:

To determine your goal **BMR** use the *Harris Benedict Formula* and insert your weight *goal* instead of your current weight. To calculate your adjusted **BMR** goal, use your goal **BMR** and adjust the number by inserting your activity level into the formula. This is the number of calories you need to limit yourself to in order to maintain your weight goal. Once you've hit your weight goal, I recommend you continue to record your total caloric intake for two or three weeks so you get an idea of the amount of food you can consume to maintain your ideal weight. I find it best to weigh once a week, Wednesday is my favorite day, to keep your weight in check. If you find you have gained a few pounds you can immediately adjust your diet or increase your exercise to take the extra weight off. If you have a hard time getting the extra pounds off, start recording everything you eat and drink again to get you back on track. Monitoring your weight closely prevents you from putting on too much weight without you knowing it. It's the best way to help you maintain your goal weight.

Knowing your numbers is an important part of attaining your weight goal and now that you know what they are, in the next chapter we'll focus on the *28 Day Plan to a Leaner, Healthier You* to help incorporate those numbers into weight loss success.

MAINTAINING YOUR WEIGHT	
Weight goal **BMR**	
Weight goal adjusted **BMR** (This is the total calories you should consume daily to maintain your weight goal.)	

CHAPTER 4
THREE SUCCESSFUL KEYS TO WEIGHT-LOSS

1. THE BEST WEIGHT-LOSS SECRET: COUNTING CALORIES

As stated earlier in this book, losing weight ultimately boils down to the amount of calories you consume and the amount of calories you burn through your daily existence and exercise. Consume more calories than you burn and you'll gain weight. Burn more calories than you consume and you'll lose weight. It's that simple! Yes, it's been discussed in this book that not all calories are equal and that four ounces of white pasta is different than four ounces of wheat pasta, but total caloric intake is still of top importance.

You now know how many calories you must restrict yourself to each day to attain your weight loss goal. Knowing how many calories you must limit yourself to is an important step, but it doesn't do you any good if you don't keep track of how many calories you consume to make sure you don't go over that number. For the examples in this book, I'll be using 1200 calories. If your caloric goal is more than this, adjust the numbers to fit your needs. (Remember, restricting your consumption to fewer than 1200 calories is NOT recommended and isn't healthy. Also, consult your physician before starting any diet program.)

To spread out your total calories, it's best to eat three small meals and two snacks per day. You can break down your total calories allowing two snacks at about 150 calories each, and then spread out the remaining 900 calories over your three main meals. (How to best do that will be under the topic "Flip-Flop Eating™.") You should have an idea of where you're going to allocate your calories throughout the day ahead of time, which makes sticking to your diet plan much easier.

The real key to keeping your caloric intake in check is to write down *everything* you eat and drink along with the calories and fat the foods contain. **This is one of the best weight loss secrets, because it really works!** If you don't record how many calories you're consuming, it's extremely difficult to govern your intake. At first this concept, might seem to be too laborious but it's actually much easier than you'd expect. Almost all products have the information you need on their nutrition facts labels and the Internet has some great websites that make finding caloric and fat content easier than ever before.

Once you get in the habit of writing down all the calories you consume, it becomes second nature. You'll even start to memorize the calories and fat content of the foods you regularly eat. You need to decide where you want to record your food intake. If you use a day planner, this is a great place to record your food consumption. You might also find it helpful to use a small notebook as a food journal that you can keep with you throughout the day, your computer or your phone. Use whatever system works best for you and your lifestyle; just make sure it's convenient so you'll stick to it. I can't emphasize enough how effective it is to write down everything you eat *and* drink. **This part of your weight loss effort is THE most important!**

To get you started on keeping a food journal and counting calories, follow the tips below to help make recording your food consumption easier.

CALORIE COUNTING MADE EASY

• **Read all food labels carefully.** Always read the nutrition facts label on the foods you consume. Keep in mind that most people consume more than a single serving of what they eat. For example, you can purchase a prepackaged snack thinking it's a single serving, when it actually can be double or even triple the serving size and you won't know it *unless* you carefully read the label. You need to become an avid label reader to know exactly how many calories and fat grams you're actually consuming.

• **Keep a measuring cup and measuring spoon readily available to measure exact amounts of food.** If you try to approximate a serving size, odds are that you'll underestimate how much you're really eating. This holds true whether you're calculating calories for brown rice or a serving of salad dressing. You need to read the labels on your food products and then measure out the exact amount of a single serving. You'll quickly find that a single serving size isn't as big as you might think.

• **Use the same bowls, cups, and plates.** This is very helpful to do because by using the same serving pieces, you'll learn where a serving or half serving falls in a particular dish. This allows you the convenience of not having to measure your food every time. I always use the same bowl for my breakfast cereal because I know exactly where a serving is in this dish. This way I know precisely how many calories I'm consuming without pulling out a measuring cup each time.

• **Utilize calorie counting websites.** For foods that don't provide nutritional labels, i.e. fruit and vegetables, calorie counting websites can be a great resource. Some websites even have the caloric information on foods from popular restaurants which is very helpful if you frequently eat out.

• **Tally the calories and fat as you prepare a meal and keep the information with the recipe for future reference.** As you mix ingredients, record the information on a note card and add up the total calories and fat grams, then divide by the amount of servings to get your per serving information. Some diet cookbooks provide this information for you making it even easier. You'll also find the recipes I've included at the end of this book helpful because the nutritional facts are listed for each one.

• **Separate your favorite snacks into single serving sizes.** At the beginning of the week. Measure out the foods you eat and separate them into re-sealable plastic bags or containers. If you do this in advance, you can quickly grab a snack and know exactly how many calories you're about to consume. Some snacks are even sold this way labeled as "100 calorie snacks." This is much more expensive than buying the food in bulk, but can offer convenience and will save you time. I don't necessarily encourage eating these pre-measured snacks because most, if not all of them, aren't the best foods for your diet effort and overall health. They tend to be high in salt and carbs without any real nutritional value to them. You're much better off separating grapes, nuts, carrots, and other healthier alternatives into single serving sizes yourself.

2. FLIP-FLOP EATING™

Flip-Flop Eating™ is all about changing *when* you eat your meals. Traditionally, we've been trained to think that breakfast should be a small meal, lunch a medium one and dinner the largest of the three. This line of thinking is actually the exact *opposite* of how your calories should be consumed. To lose weight you should "flip-flop" your meals so that your largest is early in the day and your last meal of the day is the smallest. Again, this is where the adage, "Eat breakfast like a king, lunch like a prince, and dinner like a pauper" comes into play.

Your body's metabolism typically peaks at midday and then begins to slow down. You want to eat the majority of your calories when your metabolism is at its highest to maximize the amount of calories burned. You also want to eat fewer calories when your metabolism is typically at its lowest, which is in the evening. At this time, your body slows down and will be more likely to store the food you consume instead of burning it off. For this reason, it's also recommended that you try to not eat several hours before going to bed to minimize this effect.

Flip-Flop Eating™ is a great way to enjoy some of the foods you like without sacrificing your diet effort. I personally love this concept because I have no problem eating spaghetti or chicken stir-fry for breakfast. In fact, a lot of times I'll eat a salad at night with my family and then eat the meal they had for supper as my breakfast the next morning. This way I don't feel deprived of the foods I like; I'm just eating them at a better time to help maintain my goal weight. Eating a large breakfast rich in protein helps you to feel fuller throughout the day which reduces the amount of calories you're likely to consume. Remember, breakfast is the most important meal of the day so be sure to make time to eat a healthy breakfast to get your system running again. Healthy does NOT have to mean time consuming. An apple and a handful of nuts is fast and healthy for days when you're in a rush.

TIMING IS EVERYTHING

Any carbohydrates you consume should be eaten in the earlier part of the day. Make sure the carbs are complex carbs such as whole wheat bread, brown rice, whole wheat pasta, etc. and not simple carbs. Your body does NOT need simple carbs, i.e. white bread, white pasta, white rice, or sugar. Plan your meals so your complex carbohydrates will be consumed at breakfast, for your morning snack, or lunch. After lunch, your complex carbs should be limited to what occurs naturally in non-starchy vegetables.

Fruits from the "best choice" list should be consumed early in the day due the natural sugars they contain. If you eat fruit for your afternoon snack, make sure to include a protein with it to decrease the effect of the sugar on your bloodstream. It's best, however, to try not to eat fruit after lunch if possible. This means that you need to make fruit a part of your breakfast, snack and/or lunch to ensure you get a healthy intake in your diet but time it right to help in your weight loss.

Any foods that you eat later in the day should contain a protein and a non-starchy vegetable such as broccoli, asparagus, sliced tomatoes, dark leafy greens, collards, and Brussels sprouts. Healthy, diet-friendly dinner options include combinations of salmon and asparagus, baked chicken and broccoli, or a lean cut of beef and a spinach salad. Keep the fat content low and restrict, if you can't completely eliminate, any carbohydrates.

Good meal and snack choices are laid out for you on the **28 Day Meal Schedule** but for a quick reference guide, I've listed some healthy and diet-friendly snack options below.

DIET-FRIENDLY AND HEALTHY SNACKS:
- Apple with 1 Tbsp natural peanut butter
- Lightly salted or unsalted nuts
- Low-fat cottage cheese with 1/2 serving of fruit
- 4 oz low-fat yogurt with 1 Tbsp granola or wheat germ
- 1 cup red grapes
- 1 cup of berries of choice
- 1/2 pink grapefruit
- Carrots or celery with hummus
- Mixed green salad
- 1/2 cup healthy cereal with 1/4 cup fresh or frozen blueberries
- Low-sugar oatmeal
- Hardboiled egg
- 100% whole wheat toast with low sugar jelly or hummus

3. INCREASING YOUR METABOLISM
Since the amount of calories you consume is paramount in losing weight, then it would make sense that the rate at which your body *burns* those calories, or your metabolism, would also be a critical factor. Your metabolism governs how your body burns calories and is determined by your gender, age, and genetics. If two people with different metabolic rates consume the same amount of calories and expend the same amount of physical energy, the person with the higher metabolism might lose weight while the person with the lower metabolism could maintain or even gain weight. Even though the calories consumed are the same for both people, the rate at which they burn those calories varies and creates a difference in whether they gain, maintain, or lose weight.

Your natural metabolic rate is determined by the factors mentioned above, BUT the good news is that you can take steps to help increase it. Improving your metabolism will help you tremendously in your weight loss effort. When I was younger, I used to not understand why I couldn't lose weight because I wasn't eating hardly any food. I wouldn't eat breakfast or lunch but still didn't lose weight. What I didn't realize was that my deprivation of food was hurting my efforts to lose weight because I was wrecking my metabolism. Once I started understanding the role my metabolism played in losing weight and made the necessary changes to increase it, the weight started coming off. Keep in mind that your metabolic rate naturally declines as you age so you need to make up for this fact through exercise and cutting calories. The goal is to get your metabolism as high as possible so you can burn more calories throughout the day allowing you to lose weight faster. Listed below are ways to help increase your metabolism, which will make losing weight easier.

HOW TO INCREASE YOUR METABOLISM

• **Strength training.** This is the **BEST** way to improve your metabolism! Your muscle mass is the most important factor when determining your metabolic rate because muscle burns up to *five times* the amount of calories as compared to fat. This means that for every one pound of muscle you have, you can burn up to 50 more calories per day. Therefore, if you add ten pounds of muscle mass you could burn a total of 500 more calories a day. That would help you lose a pound a week without changing anything else! You can see why this is an excellent way to aid in your weight loss effort. Strength training also has many other additional benefits which will be discussed in the next chapter.

• **Cardiovascular exercise.** Whenever you engage in any cardiovascular activity, your metabolism kicks into gear. This is a great way to speed up the calorie burning process. Even after you've stopped your cardio activity, your body will continue to burn extra calories for several more hours. On days when you can't make it into the gym or out for a walk, doing any form of movement helps increase your metabolism. There are simple things that you can do to give your metabolism a lift such as:

• *Parking near the back of a parking lot to increase your walk in the store*
• *Taking the stairs instead of the elevator*
• *Playing with your kids in the yard*
• *Vacuuming*
• *Gardening or using a push mower*
• *Running up and down the stairs in your house*
• *Walking your dog*
• *Going for a bike ride with your kids*
• *Having sex (Yet another reason to make time for you and your loved one!)*

The whole point here is to get your body moving! If you keep moving, your metabolism will keep burning those calories. It's when you're sedentary that your metabolism is signaled to slow down. Even if you're able to complete a good cardio workout in the morning, you can still do a little something in the evening to help rev up your metabolism. This will trigger your body to burn more calories helping you to lose weight faster.

• **Eat breakfast.** It's true that breakfast is the most important meal of the day. This is partly due to the reason that after a night of fasting, your body needs fuel to kick your metabolism back into gear. The word "breakfast" is exactly that – a "break" from your body's overnight "fast." As soon as you eat something your body begins to burn more calories. This also means that the sooner you eat breakfast the better because you'll start burning calories the minute food hits your system. If you don't have time for a full breakfast right when you wake up, you can still grab a couple of nuts, a yogurt, or a piece of fruit until you have the opportunity to eat a full meal. Remember to try to eat a breakfast that's high in protein and fiber to get the most out of it. Protein and fiber help you feel full which will ultimately reduce the total amount of calories you consume throughout the day. It will also give you the energy you need to get the day started.

It's a good idea to try to eat a serving of fruit for breakfast as well. This is a better time to eat something that's high in natural sugars versus eating them in the evening. You'll find it's easier to meet your recommended fruit servings per day if you can get one serving in with your breakfast meal. If you've never been a "breakfast person", it's time to change that.

If you want to lose weight and improve your overall health, start eating a healthy breakfast everyday. If you chose to skip breakfast, you're just hurting yourself because your body never revs up its metabolism which will ultimately reduce the total amount of calories you burn making losing weight more difficult.

• **Become a "grazer".** It used to be thought that snacking between meals wasn't a good thing to do, but now we know otherwise. You should eat something about every three to four hours in an effort to keep your metabolism going. As soon as your body detects that it's not receiving food regularly, it starts slowing down the rate at which it burns calories in an effort to conserve the calories your body has stored. If you eat every three to four hours, this never happens and your metabolism will continue to burn at a steady rate.

Eating frequently, or "grazing", throughout the day also helps to keep hunger at bay. It's much easier to ward off intense hunger by supplying your body with a steady flow of food than it is to satisfy your hunger once it's hit full force. Your body is meant to give you the strong urge to eat if it senses it's not getting the food it needs. Once you reach this point it's difficult to maintain the discipline to resist that urge and typically leads to binge eating or eating foods that aren't allowed on your diet plan. Keeping your body comfortably satiated improves your weight loss effort by increasing your metabolism and helps to make this diet plan a much more pleasant experience since you aren't in a constant state of hunger.

• **Drink Green Tea.** Studies have shown that green tea increases your metabolic rate while also providing your body with powerful antioxidants. Green tea is a perfect beverage to add to your diet because of the effect it has on your metabolism and for its overall health benefits. If you're used to drinking black tea and have a hard time adjusting to the flavor of green tea, try steeping two green and one black tea bag together to make it more palatable. Being from the South, it's just unnatural for me to drink tea without sugar, so I add just a little to sweeten it up. You can also try adding honey to soften its bitter flavor and for added sweetness; just make sure to include the calories in your food journal. If you don't want the caffeine, you can purchase decaffein-ated green tea but the benefits aren't as powerful as the caffeinated. As a side note, you'll be doing your children a favor if you help them develop a taste for green tea now so they receive its health benefits and continue to drink it into adulthood. Green tea doesn't have as much caffeine as black tea so you don't have to worry about your children getting hyped up just by drinking a glass a day.

• **Limit your alcohol intake.** Alcohol isn't just high in empty calories but it also slows down the rate at which your body burns fat. Alcohol consumption can sabotage your diet effort because it lowers your blood sugar levels and dehydrates your body which leads to an increase in ap-petite. So not only will you consume the extra calories contained in alcoholic beverages, but you're also likely to make poor food choices adding to your total caloric intake. To make mat-ters worse, your discipline is compromised after having a few drinks and you're likely to eat items that you normally wouldn't chose. You're also more likely to skip the next day's workout or at least not workout as intensely as you would after a night of drinking.

• **Get a good night's sleep.** Studies have shown that when you don't get the sleep your body needs there's a negative effect on the way it metabolizes carbohydrates. It also decreases the level of the hormone leptin, which sends a signal to your brain when it's full to cause you to stop eating. The decrease in this hormone leads to an increase in appetite which means an increase in calories. Another negative in sleep deprivation is that you'll decrease the likelihood of getting in a good workout the following day.

• **Drink plenty of water.** Your metabolism needs water to operate properly so make sure you consume the recommended eight, 8 ounce glasses per day. Some studies have revealed that drinking water has a very positive effect on a person's metabolism by increasing that rate at which it burns calories. Water is a very important part of your overall health and overall weight loss effort. While green tea is considered by some to be the second most perfect bev-erage for your body, water is the first. Water does more than just help you lose weight and is critical for all your bodily functions, it also improves the health and appearance of your skin, hair, and overall looks. Make drinking pure water a part of your diet plan if you don't already drink the recommended amount. There is no other beverage that can compete with this king of liquids, so make it a large part of your beverage consumption.

• **Make sure you're eating enough protein.** Protein is the building block for muscle. We dis-cussed the importance of muscle mass and its positive effect on your metabolism and in order to maximize the amount of muscle you build, you need to consume the proper amount of protein. For the typical person, it's recommended that you consume about a half of a gram of protein for every pound you weigh. So if you weigh 140 pounds you need approximately 70 grams of protein per day. Most Americans consume their required amount of protein but you still want to be aware of your intake, especially as you increase your muscle mass. As you build more muscle, you need more protein.

CHAPTER 5
28 DAYS TO A LEANER, HEALTHIER YOU

You should now be equipped with the information you need to get started on your path to weight loss, improved health, and increased energy. You can do it in 28 days if you follow this program. It's known that a person can create a habit after 21 days of repeated behavior; this plan will give you time to create new habits *and* have an extra week to spare. Twenty-eight days will also allow you to see results that will help keep you motivated to stick to your new lifestyle changes. Remember, this program is not a quick fix diet plan. It's about changing how you view food and exercise, and changing your lifestyle for good. That's what will keep you at the weight you desire and in good health. It's also what will help you have the energy you need to keep up with the demands of being a mother.

1. SETTING YOUR 28 DAY GOALS

On the chart you filled out in **Chapter 3**, you noted your weight goal. For some, this goal may be attainable in 28 days but for others it's unrealistic if you have over 8-10 pounds to lose. Even though you might not be able to reach your weight goal in exactly 28 days, you'll make great headway and will see encouraging results to keep you on track. Losing up to 2 pounds a week is a realistic and safe weight loss goal. (Some diets claim you can lose a lot more than this, but most aren't very credible and people usually tend to quickly gain back any weight they lose.) How much you're able to lose per week for the first 28 days depends on your initial weight, as well as how many calories you cut and the amount of physical activity in which you participate. Someone who needs to lose 50 pounds will drop weight faster than someone who only needs to lose only five.

Take this information into account when deciding what your 28 day weight-loss goal is going to be. Don't set yourself up with an unrealistic goal just to be let down causing you to get discouraged. Make your goal one you need to work for yet is attainable. Set a reward for yourself once you've reached your goal in the 28 days. A reward does not mean food. I'm referring to treating yourself to a facial, massage, new pair of shoes, outfit, etc. Don't view food as a reward. Adding something to your wardrobe is a long lasting reward, and treating yourself to a massage or facial is a great way to relax and recharge. If you have an outfit your been wanting, take a picture of it and post it on your refrigerator to help motivate you. These types of rewards, unlike treating yourself to a fancy dinner, won't sabotage your diet effort. If you're on a tight budget, think of the money you saved by eating less and not eating fast food or other costly junk food. You've worked hard to lose the weight and you deserve to be rewarded!

Record your 28 day goals on the chart below. Make a copy of your goals and post them in a place where you'll see them frequently such as your refrigerator. Posting your weight goal on the refrigerator is a very helpful way to prevent you from eating foods that aren't a part of your food plan. I've personally found this to be very effective. You can add even more motivation by putting up a picture of someone that you view as being in great shape. (I've done this in the past and I used to laugh when my younger kids would always want to know who the lady on the refrigerator was.) Writing down goals and having them visible has been proven to be effective in helping people attain the goals they set in every aspect of life. Write your goals down in your planner, on your bathroom mirror, in your car, on your phone or computer home screen, or wherever you need so you stay focused on what you're trying to accomplish.

Record your information on the chart below and leave the goals for cardio and strength training blank until you've read **Chapter 7** which discusses exercise. Once you've read it, come back and fill in your workout goals.

28 DAY GOALS:	
Current weight:	28 Day weight goal:
Total weight to lose in 28 days:	
Days for cardio work:	Days for strength training:
Reward:	

2. ALLOCATING YOUR CALORIES:

Take your total calories you're allowed to consume to reach your goal as calculated in Chapter 3 and divide them out among your three main meals and two snacks. Use the example below as a guide to see the best way to spread out your calories. Remember, this book uses 1200 calories when tracking calorie distribution. If your caloric intake is higher than this, adjust your numbers accordingly. This is also an estimation of caloric intake and you can be flexible within this chart. The key is to make sure that most of your calories are to be consumed early in the day and then taper off as the day progresses.

1200 CALORIES:		
MEAL	**TIME OF DAY**	**CALORIES ALLOWED**
Breakfast	6:00 AM	300
Snack	9:00 AM	200
Lunch	12:30 PM	275
Snack	3:30 PM	200
Dinner	6:30 PM	225

3. YOUR 28 DAY MEAL SCHEDULE

Snacks should generally consist of around 150-200 calories each depending on how you allocate your calories throughout the day. The two snacks you eat each day should be a nutritious addition to your diet and give you the opportunity to keep your blood sugar stable, keep your metabolism revved up, and help keep hunger at bay. Don't allow your snacks to be a free-for-all. The amount of calories you consume still needs to be monitored so you don't consume too many. Sometimes dieters who aren't careful let "grazing" backfire because they eat more calories at each meal or snack than allowed. This is why it's so important to write down everything you eat so you know exactly how many calories you're consuming.

Follow the **28 Day Meal Schedule** to help get you on the fast track to weight loss. For each day you'll find three meals and two snacks based on a caloric intake of 1200 calories. If you choose to consume more calories, add it to each meal or snack proportionately. Remember that you want to consume most of your calories earlier in the day while keeping your last meal small and without starchy carbohydrates.

For the meals listed, I use extra-lean ground turkey instead of beef. If you prefer to use red meat buy the leanest you can find and drain out any grease by placing several layers of paper towels on top of newspaper, spread the meat on top, cover with more paper towels and press firmly to extract as much grease as possible. If you don't eat a particular group of food that I've mentioned, just substitute other meal suggestions in its place. The recipes and snacks in the meal schedule that are marked with an asterisk can be found in Chapter 9. You can also refer to the additional recipes in Chapter 9 and incorporate them into your 28 day menu. Make sure to calculate the caloric information listed after each recipe so you still keep your total caloric intake for the day at 1200. I understand that people have different likes and dislikes as well as food allergies, so make adjustments accordingly to fit your needs. It's important, however, to be open-minded about trying new foods which you might discover you really like. This will make the transition to your new healthier lifestyle easier and more enjoyable.

BEFORE YOU BEGIN:
FEED YOUR FAMILY AND STILL LOSE WEIGHT WITH ONE MEAL

Our children need to consume more good carbs and good fats than we do. It's important to learn how to make meals work for your diet efforts while providing your family with all the nutrients they need to support their active and growing bodies. This isn't as challenging as you might think. You can plan healthy meals for your family and make them a part of your diet by eating smaller portions of what you serve them and leaving out the carbohydrates or high fat items your family eats.

In the **28 Day Meal Schedule**, you can take the meal suggestions from the charts and then add the appropriate rice or pasta dish for your family to eat. This allows you and your family to eat the same entrée and vegetable with you just adding an extra side dish for them that you don't consume. This allows you to cook one meal that keeps you on your diet plan and offers your family a healthy dinner, with all the calories and nutrients they need.

For example, when the meal schedule calls for a turkey burger with steamed broccoli you just eat the burger *without* the bun. For your family, you can also add baked sweet potato fries, corn on the cob, baked beans, etc. When the meal calls for salmon and asparagus, everyone gets to eat the entrée and vegetable, all you have to do is add a pasta dish or wild rice for the rest of the family to complete the meal. Tacos are another example of this because your family gets a traditional easy taco meal and you can eat it too – just leave out the cheese and taco shells, and of course use lean ground turkey or beef and squeeze out any grease as discussed previously. The goal is to minimize your effort by preparing one meal that everyone can eat, yet still allow you to lose weight. Your whole family will benefit from your new healthier way of eating and it will create good eating habits that will stay with them throughout their lives.

The **28 Day Program** is simply two weeks of meals and snacks planned out for you to make your weight loss and lifestyle change easier. You repeat the menus after the end of day 14 to give you the full 28 days. You'll also find the recommended cardiovascular and strength training schedule which will be discussed in more detail in **Chapter 6 – Creating a Workout Program.**

This will give you a solid game plan on when you should strength train and how much cardio you should be doing. I planned out this schedule to make achieving your goals simple. If you choose not to follow the meal plan, just make sure your keeping your caloric intake at the number you calculated to reach your goals. Your success will increase however, if you know ahead of time what you'll be eating and what you need to shop for. This **28 Day Program** helps take all the guess work out of losing weight and is easy to follow. *Please note that the caloric and fat calculated for each meal and snack is an estimation. Some days the daily menu might be below the 1200 calories but you can add in an additional caloric beverage or food to make up for the calories to bring you to 1200. Those are calories of your choice that you can add in your daily intake. Now all you need to do is read through the menus, make your grocery list, hit the store and start your* **28 Days To a Leaner, Healthier You!**

DAY 1

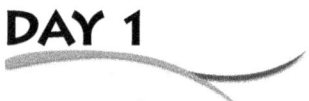

		CALORIES	FAT
BREAKFAST:	6 oz Greek Yogurt with 1 Tbsp wheat germ. 10 mixed almonds. Coffee, tea or water	200	5
SNACK:	1 apple with 1 Tbsp peanut butter	155	8
LUNCH:	100% whole wheat bread (1 slice) with hummus or Tuna Salad*, lettuce & tomato	200	5
SNACK:	MC's Heart-Healthy Salad*, 1 boiled egg	130	7
DINNER:	Turkey burger* (1/2 of whole wheat bun), 1/2 cup Steamed Broccoli*	250	3
TOTAL:		935	28
CARDIO:	15 minutes (5 warm up, 10 post workout)		
STRENGTH TRAINING:	30 minutes, full body with stretching		

DAY 2

		CALORIES	FAT
BREAKFAST:	1 cup of whole grain cereal, 1 cup skim or almond milk with 1/4 cup frozen or fresh blueberries. Coffee, tea or water	270	2
SNACK:	*Kashi TLC Bar, Fiber One Bar, Zone Bar,* or the like	150	5
LUNCH:	Turkey sandwich on 1 slice of whole wheat bread, mustard, lettuce, tomato, mozzarella cheese stick, 8 baby carrots	235	8
SNACK:	6 oz Greek Yogurt , 1 oz granola	280	7
DINNER:	MC's Heart-Healthy Salad with Chicken strips*	145	4
TOTAL:		1080	26
CARDIO:	30 minutes		
STRENGTH TRAINING:	Rest		

DAY 3

		CALORIES	FAT
BREAKFAST:	1 slice 100% whole wheat bread with 1/2 Tbsp jelly, 1 egg, 1 cup of skim or almond milk. Coffee, hot tea or water	235	6
SNACK:	1/2 cup low or fat-free cottage cheese, 1/2 cup fruit of choice	135	3
LUNCH:	MC's Heart-Healthy Salad*, 7 walnut halves	160	13
SNACK:	Apple, 1 Tbsp peanut butter	155	8
DINNER:	3 oz boiled shrimp (or baked chicken), Stir-Fried Carrots*, 1/2 cup brown rice	310	5
TOTAL:		955	35
CARDIO:	25 minutes *(5 warm up, 20 post work out)*		
STRENGTH TRAINING:	30 minutes full body with stretching		

DAY 4

		CALORIES	FAT
BREAKFAST:	1 1/2 cup Perfect Smoothie*, 10 mixed nuts. Coffee, tea or water	180	6
SNACK:	*Kashi TLC Bar, Fiber One Bar, Zone Bar*, or the like	150	5
LUNCH:	1 cup skim milk, hummus or Tuna Salad on whole wheat bread*, lettuce & tomato, 1 fruit of choice	370	3
SNACK:	MC's Heart-Healthy Salad*, 1/2 cup low-fat cottage cheese	160	5
DINNER:	3 oz Filet Mignon or flank steak, Steamed Asparagus* and sliced tomatoes	225	9
TOTAL:		1085	28
CARDIO:	Rest		
STRENGTH TRAINING:	Rest		

DAY 5

		CALORIES	FAT
BREAKFAST:	1/2 dry cup plain oatmeal (cooked) with 1/2 cup fruit. Coffee, tea or water	185	3
SNACK:	6 oz Greek Yogurt	140	0
LUNCH:	1 slice 100% whole wheat bread with hummus or Tuna Salad*, lettuce & tomato, carrots or celery sticks	200	3
SNACK:	1 cup red grapes, 1 oz mixed nuts	290	15
DINNER:	Baked Parmesan Salmon*, 1/2 cup brown rice, Steamed Broccoli*	165	12
TOTAL:		980	33
CARDIO:	30 minutes *(5 warm up, 25 post workout)*		
STRENGTH TRAINING:	30 minutes, full body with stretching		

DAY 6

		CALORIES	FAT
BREAKFAST:	2 eggs, 1 slice 100% whole wheat bread with 1/2 Tbsp jelly, 1 cup skim or almond milk. Coffee, tea or water	305	10
SNACK:	6 oz Greek Yogurt, 1/4 cup blueberries	160	0
LUNCH:	1 serving Spaghetti with Meat Sauce*	280	3
SNACK:	*Kashi TLC Bar, Fiber One Bar, Zone Bar,* or the like	150	5
DINNER:	Tuscan Pork Roast*, Stir-Fry Broccoli*	300	13
TOTAL:		1195	31
CARDIO:	25-35 minutes fun activity with stretching. *(bike riding with the kids, tennis, roller blading, fast walking, etc.)*		
STRENGTH TRAINING:	Rest		

DAY 7

		CALORIES	FAT
BREAKFAST:	1 serving plain oatmeal with 1/3 cup Craisins. Coffee, tea or water	280	3
SNACK:	1 cup red grapes, 10 almonds	290	15
LUNCH:	Power Vegetable Soup*	145	1
SNACK:	MC's Heart-Healthy Salad*	60	3
DINNER:	Slow-Cooked Chicken*, Brussels sprouts*, 1/2 cup brown rice	275	3
TOTAL:		1050	25
CARDIO:	Rest		
STRENGTH TRAINING:	Rest		

DAY 8

		CALORIES	FAT
BREAKFAST:	1⁄2 whole wheat bagel with 1/2 Tbsp low fat cream cheese, 1⁄2 pink grapefruit. Coffee, tea or water	135	4
SNACK:	1 oz mixed nuts, 1 cup strawberries or blueberries	260	15
LUNCH:	Slow-Cooked Chicken*, Steamed Asparagus*, 1⁄2 cup whole wheat pasta	360	3
SNACK:	Carrot or celery sticks with hummus	90	4
DINNER:	Power Vegetable Soup*, small salad	180	2
TOTAL:		1025	28
CARDIO:	25 minutes, *(5 warm up, 20 post workout)*		
STRENGTH TRAINING:	35 minutes, full body with stretching		

DAY 9

		CALORIES	FAT
BREAKFAST:	1 1⁄2 cup Perfect Smoothie, 7 walnut halves. Coffee, tea or water	180	6
SNACK:	1⁄2 pink grapefruit, 10 mixed nuts	120	6
LUNCH:	1 slice whole wheat bread with Tuna Salad* or hummus, lettuce and tomato, mozzarella stick, carrot sticks	280	9
SNACK:	1 apple, 1 Tbsp peanut butter	155	8
DINNER:	Tex-Mex Turkey Tenderloin*, Steamed Asparagus*, 1⁄2 cup brown rice	310	2
TOTAL:		1045	31
CARDIO:	35 minutes with stretching		
STRENGTH TRAINING:	Rest		

DAY 10

		CALORIES	FAT
BREAKFAST:	6 oz Greek Yogurt, 1 oz granola	280	7
SNACK:	1 cup of whole grain cereal, 1 cup skim milk, 1/4 cup berries	270	2
LUNCH:	Tex-Mex Turkey Tenderloin*, Steamed Asparagus*, 1/2 cup brown rice	310	2
SNACK:	MC's Heart-Healthy Salad*	60	3
DINNER:	3 oz boiled shrimp, Simple Sautéed Mushrooms and Onions*	150	3
TOTAL:		1070	17
CARDIO:	25 minutes, (5 warm up, 20 post workout)		
STRENGTH TRAINING:	35 minutes, full body with stretching		

DAY 11

		CALORIES	FAT
BREAKFAST:	1 cup of whole grain cereal , 1 cup skim or almond milk with 1/4 cup frozen or fresh blueberries. Coffee, tea or water	270	2
SNACK:	1 apple and 10 mixed nuts	150	6
LUNCH:	MC's Heart-Healthy Salad* topped with 3 oz boiled shrimp, 1 cup red grapes	245	4
SNACK:	Celery sticks with hummus	90	4
DINNER:	Honey Mustard Chicken*, Sautéed Squash and Zucchini*	195	6
TOTAL:		950	22
CARDIO:	Rest		
STRENGTH TRAINING:	Rest		

DAY 12

		CALORIES	FAT
BREAKFAST:	1 slice 100% whole wheat bread with 1/2 Tbsp jelly, 1 egg. Coffee, tea or water	235	6
SNACK:	1 apple with 1 Tbsp peanut butter	155	8
LUNCH:	1 cup Power Vegetable Soup* and small salad	205	4
SNACK:	6 oz Greek Yogurt, 1/4 cup blueberries	170	0
DINNER:	Pineapple-Chicken Rice Bake*	280	3
TOTAL:		1045	21
CARDIO:	30 minutes *(5 warm up, 25 post workout)*		
STRENGTH TRAINING:	30 minutes, full body with stretching		

DAY 13

		CALORIES	FAT
BREAKFAST:	1 1/2 cup Perfect Smoothie*, 10 almonds. Coffee, tea or water	180	6
SNACK:	*Kashi TLC Bar, Fiber One Bar, Zone Bar,* or the like	150	5
LUNCH:	Turkey sandwich on 1 slice 100% whole wheat bread, mustard, lettuce, tomato, carrot sticks	155	2
SNACK:	1/2 red grapefruit, 10 mixed nuts	100	5
DINNER:	Scallops with Linguine*, Steamed Asparagus*	360	7
TOTAL:		945	25
CARDIO:	25-35 fun activity with stretching. *(Bike riding with kids, tennis, roller blading)*		
STRENGTH TRAINING:	Rest		

DAY 14

		CALORIES	FAT
BREAKFAST:	1 serving oatmeal with 1⁄2 cup strawberries. Coffee, tea or water	185	3
SNACK:	6 oz Greek Yogurt	140	0
LUNCH:	3 oz baked chicken breast, Broccoli and Pasta with Onion Sauce*	215	4
SNACK:	1 oz mixed nuts	170	15
DINNER:	Chicken Marsala*, 1⁄2 cup brown rice, small salad	340	7
TOTAL:		1050	29
CARDIO:	Rest		
STRENGTH TRAINING:	35 minutes, full body with stretching		

SIDE NOTES:

• You'll notice the same meals are repeated within a day or two of each other. This help you save on time by maximizing leftovers so you spend less time in the kitchen.

• All nuts should be low-sodium or no-salt mixes. Walnuts, Brazil nuts, almonds, pine nuts, cashews, pecans, hazelnuts, pistachios and macadamias are the best while peanuts are the least desirable. If you're unable to find low-salt mixes, mix the contents of salted and unsalted nuts to reduce the total salt content. If you have a nut allergy and are soy tolerant, substitute soy nuts when the meal plan calls for nuts.

• If you add sugar, milk or cream to your coffee or tea, remember to add this to your total caloric intake. The milk should be fat-free and if you must use cream make sure it's low-fat or fat-free.

• If you drink *V8* and tomato juice they should be reduced sodium. The regular versions of these juices are very high in sodium.

• The peanut butter you choose should not contain partially hydrogenated oils. Look for labels that state "non-hydrogenated" or "natural". Almond butter is even a better choice and many brands have no sodium or added ingredients; their only ingredient is almonds.

• For snacks that mention granola, you can purchase plain granola or crunch up all natural granola bars such as *Nature's Own*, and ration the bars over several snacks. I like using granola bars because they're snacks that my children love too. Just make sure not to use too much because they have a high sugar content.

• Whenever fruit is mentioned, your best choices are the ones with the most color. Grapefruit should be pink and not white. Grapes should be red and not green, onions red and not yellow, etc. The more color in your produce, the better it is for you.

• When using seafood, always choose wild caught and not farmed raised. Farmed raised seafood may not contain the same health benefits and can have high levels of environmental contaminants. Buying seafood from the US is a much better choice than seafood caught in other countries, so pay attention to its origin as well.

• Always cook with poultry that's skinless. If you opt to purchase poultry with the skin on to help save on your food bill, make sure to remove it prior to cooking.

• Always cook with extra virgin olive oil which is the healthiest. Your second choice should be canola oil. You can also use cooking sprays that are canola or olive oil based.

THE IMPORTANCE OF EXERCISE

Cutting calories isn't the only thing you need to do to lose weight; you also have to exercise. In the 28 day schedule listed above, exercise is incorporated in on most days. Following an exercise program is an important part of successful weight loss and maintenance and a person who sticks with an exercise program will lose weight faster and increase her odds of keeping it off for good. Even if you can reach your weight goal just by cutting calories, it can't compare to the look and feel you'll have by strengthening your body through cardiovascular activity and strength training.

Losing fat is the goal but it's much better to replace the fat with muscle. Developing muscles gives the appearance a person is slimmer than she really is because there's more definition to the body. In fact, even if you don't lose weight but develop more muscles, you'll look slimmer. Aiding in weight loss and physical appearance aren't the only reasons to make working out a part of your life. Your overall health will improve in the short and long run, *and* you'll find that your energy level will increase. I know every mom could use that!

Listed below are just a few of the many reasons why working out is so important and should become a part of your lifestyle no matter how busy you are. Read the list of benefits and you'll be convinced exercise is a necessary part of living a healthy life.

BENEFITS OF EXERCISE:
• Lose weight faster
• Improve the odds of keeping off the weight you lose
• Reduce the risks of chronic diseases such as certain types of cancer, osteoporosis, type 2 diabetes, and heart disease
• Strengthen your heart and lungs
• Reduce the risk of premature death
• Reduce depression and anxiety
• Improve your mood
• Promote better sleep
• Improve your sex life
• Build and maintain healthy muscles, bones, and joints
• Improve coordination and balance
• Feel more confident
• Look toned and healthy

I know we're all extremely busy with everything that's going on in our lives, but the list above should be enough for you to realize you *have* to take time out to exercise. I love the saying that "if you don't take the time to exercise, then you'll have to take the time to be sick." This is so true. You brush your teeth daily to keep them clean and healthy just like you wash your hair and body. It's just something you know you have to do, so you do it. The rest of your body deserves the same attention. Exercising is not just about your weight, it's about your health!

The title of this book is **Lose Weight, Feel Great!**, and exercising is one of the main ways to help you accomplish both. You have to make working out a priority in your life no matter how difficult it might seem at first. Start scheduling in your workout sessions like you would a doctor's appointment so you know you're committed to that time. Finding the time to exercise with the demands of being a mother might not be easy at first but the benefits of it outweigh the efforts it takes to make it happen. If you have a full schedule, you just have to get creative about how to fit exercise into your life. Read the following ideas on fitting exercise into your routine and find the one that best suits your lifestyle and the ages of your children.

How to Find Time to Exercise

• If your children are still young and not in school or you work during the day and can't get to the gym, start waking up before your family to workout. I along with a lot of other mothers, have found great success in doing this. I used to set my alarm for 5:00am so I could get to the gym or go for a run and be home before anyone in the house woke up. I was still able to serve breakfast and get everyone out the door to school or work without them even knowing I was ever gone. (I know this is understood, but only do this if your spouse or another adult is in the house.) I loved the fact that I had created this time to workout and nothing else I did during the day had to be compromised. The time might seem early to you at first, but you'll find that exercising will give you more energy in the long run and help you sleep better at night. The early morning is a perfect time to follow my workout program because you don't need fancy workout equipment and you won't lose time driving to and from a gym. If you don't own any cardio machines, you can simply jump rope, do jumping jacks or rent or buy a DVD geared to get your heart rate up before performing the strength exercises.

• If your children are of stroller age, invest in a good jogging stroller and walk or run with your children in tow. If you time it around their nap it increases your odds of a successful outing. After your walk or run, leave your children in the stroller while you do your strength training workout outside with them. (I used to keep an extra set of dumbbells in the garage just for this purpose.) If they're awake when you get back to the house, you can still workout in front of them. Try counting your reps out loud or have them count for you to keep them entertained. You can also let them play outside while you complete your strength training routine.

• Purchase one pound dumbbells for your children so they can workout with you. Children love this and it'll help foster a love for exercising they'll carry with them throughout their lives. *(My father did this with my brother and me by lifting weights after work. He made us our own weight bar and we would work out with him and run sprints even as young children. The love of working out has stuck with us both ever since.)*

• If you work outside the home, schedule in a workout during your lunch hour. Even just a 15-20 minute walk is beneficial if that's all you can fit in. If you join a gym that's close by you can work out and take a quick shower if needed. Even if your lunch hour doesn't allow time for a good workout, you might consider going right before work or immediately afterwards before you head home or pick up the kids.

• In the evening or at night after your children are asleep, exercise to a workout DVD or utilize a tread mill or any other piece of exercise equipment you might have. If you watch TV, this is the perfect opportunity to make better use of your viewing time. Be aware however, that if you exercise at night it's very easy to miss a workout if you've had a long day at work or with the kids. When you exercise in the morning you tend to be fresher and more likely to stick to your commitment.

• Find an exercise partner to workout with. This helps you stay motivated because working out with a partner adds extra accountability that you might not feel if you're working out by yourself. Some people find it harder to let others down than it is to let themselves down. An exercise buddy is also a perfect motivator for someone who is prone to procrastinate. Another benefit of working out with someone is the social aspect. It's more fun to workout when you can visit and have fun being with a friend.

• If your children are old enough, get your walk or run in while your family rides bikes. You can even help your children develop a love of running by allowing them to run with you. This is a great time to share together and a bonding experience that can stay with you throughout your life. Running as a family can be beneficial in more ways that just to get exercise. If you can get your children in on your exercise routine early, you will *all* reap the rewards.

• Workout with your spouse. This can be a great way to bond as a couple while getting you both healthy and in shape. You can take turns pushing the jogging stroller or try to fit in a workout while the children are in school.

• If you can afford to hire a trainer, do it! Having a personal trainer to teach and motivate you can pay off immediately and down the road. I hired a trainer that I worked with during my 3rd pregnancy and after delivery. I *still* benefit and use what I learned from him to this day. It seemed costly at the time, but I definitely got my money's worth because I still apply what I learned and I lost all the baby weight in three months. The key to making the most out of your trainer is to write down your exercise routine or make sure you remember what exercise moves you learn, so you can continue to do them long after you've stopped paying for the trainer. Now as a trainer myself, I encourage my clients to do the same so they keep their momentum going long after our training sessions have completed.

• You can also take advantage of my online personal training at www.todaysbalancedmom.com. The various packages available are a great way to stay motivated, get educated on health, fitness and diet and also have the opportunity to get personalized instruction and feedback to help you reach your goals.

You've seen all the benefits of exercising and some ideas to help you incorporate it into your life so now it's time to get you started on your workout program. If you've never had an exercise regime before, don't worry. This program works for anyone whether they have a history of working out or not. Those who have never exercised regularly can quickly get accustomed to the routine. If you have always exercised, you can simply add time to the cardio and/or intensity of the strength training based on your fitness level. Make it a top priority to stick with the program for the 28 days and you'll quickly find that it gets increasingly easier to make the time to workout. You'll even discover that you start to crave exercise if you ever have to miss a workout. At first you might view working out as something you *have* to do, but you'll soon see it as something you *want* to do. You'll also likely discover that you're ready to add more time and intensity to your routine and/or increase the frequency you participate in it. *(Always remember, however, that you **must** take a day's rest between weight sessions so your body can recover. The exception to this is if you strength train your upper body one day and then work your lower body the next. You just don't want to work the same muscle group two days in a row. Also, be sure to check with your physician before starting any exercise routine.)*

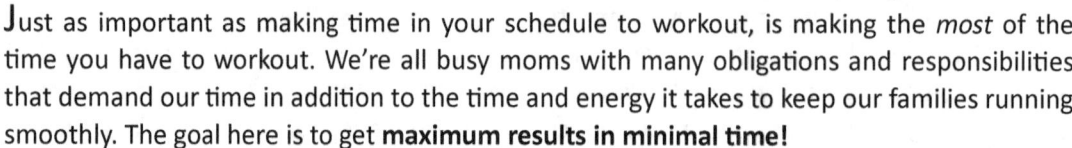

CHAPTER 6
MAXIMUM RESULTS IN MINIMAL TIME
CREATING AN EFFECTIVE WORKOUT PROGRAM

Just as important as making time in your schedule to workout, is making the *most* of the time you have to workout. We're all busy moms with many obligations and responsibilities that demand our time in addition to the time and energy it takes to keep our families running smoothly. The goal here is to get **maximum results in minimal time!**

There are plenty of people who put a lot of time and energy into their workout routine but don't get the results they want. Just like you have to eat smart to attain your weight goal, you have to workout smart to get the body you want. You can workout in less time and get better results by working out effectively.

This chapter will show you how to get the most out of the time you spend exercising. Cardio-vascular activity, strength training and flexibility are the three major components of exercise and will be discussed individually. An important key to remember when you're working out is that it *is* work. You have to push yourself and challenge your body to get the results you desire. After you've completed each workout, you should feel like you've given it your all. When engaging in a cardio activity carrying on a conversation should be somewhat difficult. If you're able to easily chat with someone, you're not working hard enough. You should expect to be sore after a workout. Consider your soreness reassurance that you've pushed your body and are on the road to getting the results you want. Keep in mind that there is a difference from being sore and injuring your muscles or joints. You should feel the burn of your muscle as you work it but you should never be in pain. If you do feel pain in a certain area, you need to take a break from that particular activity until the pain subsides. Applying ice packs on the sore area and taking an anti-inflammatory will help speed up the healing process allowing you to get back into your routine sooner.

1. CARDIOVASCULAR ACTIVITY:

For the cardio portion of your workout routine, you can choose from a variety of activities. Whichever activity appeals to you is fine as long as it keeps your heart rate elevated. Different activities affect your heart rate in different ways, so increase the intensity if you're heart rate isn't as high as it should be. An easy way to gauge this is the conversation rule. If you can easily carry on a conversation while participating in cardio activity, you need to speed it up. A casual stroll isn't going to help you reach your goals. It needs to be a fast walk to get your heart pumping. The more intense the activity, the more calories you'll burn. For this workout program, cardio activity is recommended before each strength training session. You can also get an additional burst of fat burning by completing some form of intense cardio work after you strength train.

On days that you don't strength train, participating in any form of cardio work is recommended. The more cardio you fit into your schedule, the faster you'll get the results you want. Even if you only fit in 15 minutes of an activity, it's better than not doing anything. A lot of people have the misconception that if they can't get in a full workout it's not worth the effort. This isn't true. Doing *anything* is better than doing nothing. At the end of the evening, a brisk 10 minute walk burns extra calories and revs up your metabolism. Also, just engaging in housework or gardening at the end of the day will have a positive effect on calories burned and your metabolism - so will sex! If it gets your heart pumping, you'll benefit.

Mixing up the cardio activity you participate in helps keep your body guessing and maximizes your workout. Vary your cardio exercise to help your body work different areas. This also prevents you from getting bored with the same routine and can help prevent injuries. You can also incorporate interval training into your workout routine to keep it interesting and to get great results fast by increasing the amount of fat you burn.

Incorporating interval training is a fun and effective way to mix up your routine. Interval training is the change of intensity of your aerobic activity for brief intervals that range from 15 seconds to 5 minutes. First you participate in an aerobic activity at a moderate pace then dramatically increase the intensity for a short period of time, and then slow it down for an "active" recovery. You can use interval training with any cardiovascular workout including walking, running, swimming, rowing or biking. According to many experts, interval training is more effective in burning fat and strengthening your heart than just maintaining a steady pace throughout your workout. In fact, it's been proven that 20 minutes of interval training can have the same health benefits of 40 minutes of cardio at a steady pace. It's perfect for when you're short on time and it also mixes things up a bit to keep you from getting bored.

AN EXAMPLE OF INTERVAL TRAINING COULD LOOK SOMETHING LIKE THIS:

· *Walk for 4 minutes*
· *Run for 1 minute*
· *Return to your walking speed for 4 more minutes*
· *Repeat these steps for 30 minutes*

As your fitness level increases, you can add to the intensity of the workout and/or increase the duration. Interval training is a great way to get the most out of your workout by helping you to burn extra fat and calories while also strengthening your heart. One of my favorite ways to interval train when I'm on a treadmill is to walk at a good pace for five minutes and then increase the incline dramatically and walk backwards for 1-2 minutes. (I definitely recommend holding onto the side rails while doing this to prevent a wipe out.) Turn around and reduce the incline and resume your pace for five minutes and repeat. You will get a great workout doing this and it makes it fun and different. The more creative you get with your workouts, the more you'll enjoy them and the more likely you are to stick to your workout routine.

To give you an idea of calories burned per activity look at the list below of different activities and the amount of calories burned for each.

ACTIVITY	CALORIES BURNED PER HOUR
Walking *(20 minute miles)*	300
Walking *(15 minute miles)*	350
Running *(12 minute miles)*	575
Running *(10 minute miles)*	685
Bicycling *(5.5 miles/hour)*	450
Bicycling *(10 miles/hour)*	700
Elliptical *(moderate)*	300
Elliptical *(intense)*	700
Rollerblading	420
Swimming *(intense)*	500
Step Aerobics *(moderate)*	550
Step Aerobics *(advanced step)*	700
Pilates *(moderate)*	300
Yoga *(standard form)*	400
Tai Chi *(moderate)*	400
Basic Aerobics	450
Strength training *(moderate)*	215
Strength training *(intense)*	430
Tennis *(moderate singles)*	450
Tennis *(intense singles)*	650
Golf *(with cart)*	180
Golf *(without cart)*	240

* This chart is based on a 150 pound woman. To find calories burned per hour for your weight, take the number listed and divide by 60 minutes. Then divide by 150 lbs. Take your answer and multiply by your own weight in pounds and again by the minutes of activity.

2. STRENGTH TRAINING:

We discussed briefly the important role strength training plays in reaching your weight goal due to its positive effect on your metabolism. We have learned that the more muscle you have, the more calories you burn just through daily existence - up to five times the amount. Adding muscle mass to your body is key to effective weight loss.

A lot of females have a preconceived misconception about strength training. Many women have avoided lifting weights for fear they'll "bulk up." It goes against the nature of the female body to bulk up. You would have to engage in extremely intense weight lifting to get the bulk that so many women have been afraid of. The real fear should be having a body without *any* muscle tone. Our society is starting to change its view on women and strength training as more and more women are seeing the advantages of increasing their muscle tone. The benefits of strength training are amazing. Read through the list below and you'll quickly see why strength training is an important part of your exercise regimen.

BENEFITS:

- Increases metabolic rate
- Prevents osteoporosis
- Increases muscle mass while decreasing fat
- Improves strength, power and endurance
- Improves balance, coordination, flexibility, mobility and stability
- Prevents injuries by strengthening muscles and joints
- Reduces risk of coronary disease
- Lowers cholesterol and blood pressure
- Reduces risk of adult onset diabetes
- Reduces risk of colon cancer
- Lowers resting heart rate
- Improves the function of immune system
- Improves posture
- Prevents lower back injuries
- Improves glucose tolerance and insulin sensitivity
- Aids in rehabilitation and recovery by strengthening muscles surrounding injured area
- Enhanced performance in sports and exercise
- Improves mood
- Helps you look and feel great!

3. FLEXIBILITY

This is one of the most forgotten components of an effective workout routine. Unfortunately, many people neglect to stretch after a workout because they don't understand it's importance. Stretching improves flexibility, athletic performance and reduces the risk of injury. It also increases the blood flow to your muscles and improves your range of motion.

When you stretch, do NOT bounce. Gently stretch your muscles to a point where you feel it but it's not painful. Hold each stretch for 20-30 seconds. Five minutes of stretching is all you need to reap the benefits.

Strength Training Exercises:

The exercises on the following pages can easily be done at home with just a set of dumbbells. If you don't own hand weights you can purchase them without making a huge financial investment. They can be found at sporting goods stores, large discount chain stores and you can get an even better price at sport stores that sell used equipment. Try out a couple of weights to find the ones that will be good for you. I recommend getting two sets because you will probably want different poundage for different moves. A set of 5 to 8 pound and a set of 10 to 12 pound dumbbells would be a good start. Try them out in the store to see what's comfortable for you. Later you might need to increase the weight as your strength improves. For each move you should be able to complete at least 8 repetitions. If you can't, you need to decrease the weight amount. If you can *easily* complete 15 reps with a particular weight you need to increase the poundage.

It's very important to maintain proper form while lifting weights in order to get the most out of the exercise *and* to prevent injuries. Lifting weights in front of a mirror is an excellent way to ensure you're using good form. Listed below are a few standard guidelines to lifting properly:

1. *Keep your head and shoulders up, with your shoulders in line with your hips.*
2. *Knees should be slightly bent during upper body exercises to take the stress off your back.*
3. *Exhale during the most difficult part of the exercise. Never hold your breath!*
4. *Your knees should never extend past your toes when performing leg exercises.*
5. *Keep movements controlled and slow.*
6. *Stretch each muscle group you work to help release the tension.*
7. *Wear cushioned shoes to give your body support.*

In the next section you'll find the recommended strength training moves to target each part of your body. Start this routine only after engaging in some form of cardio activity. Follow the **28 Day Schedule** in **Chapter 5** to get you started. After completing your cardio, start with your legs then work your arms and lastly, your abdominal muscles and core. Stick to this order but occasionally mix up the moves within a certain muscle group to create "muscle confusion" to get better results. Slow controlled movements will give you the best benefit from each exercise, so don't rush through your routine. You'll get the most out of each move if you perform slow movements even when returning to your start position. Some people will make the mistake of controlling their movement only on the front end of the exercise, and then quickly return to the start position. Get maximum results by maintaining slow movement through the *entire* exercise. One last important tip before you get started is you should **ALWAYS** give your body a day of rest between weight lifting sessions. This is when your muscles recover which is critical to getting results and preventing injuries.

Work through this routine on the days designated for strength training. Take it easy the first week and focus mostly on using the correct form instead of trying to lift a heavier weight or do more reps. Proper form is important in getting the most out of your workout. Once you know you're executing the moves correctly, add reps or more weight as needed.

LOWER BODY

LUNGES

- Stand with feet shoulder-width apart and hands on hips.
- Lunge forward with one leg, bending knee until thigh is parallel to the floor.
- Do not let your knee extend past your toes.
- Make sure the heel of your front foot remains on the floor.

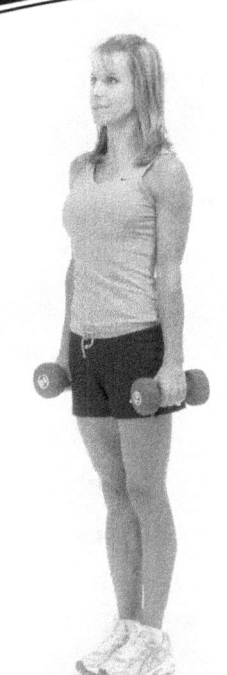

2

- Return your leg to the starting position and repeat with the same leg.

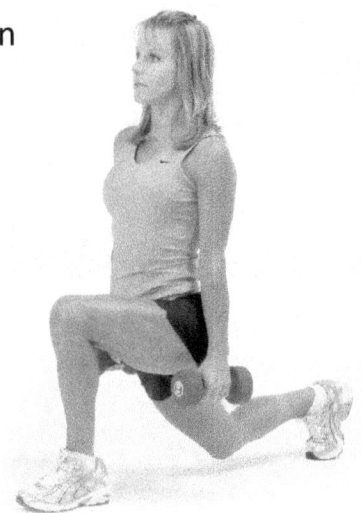

BEGINNER:
- Complete a set of 15 reps per leg

ADVANCED:
- Add 5-15 pound dumbbells and complete 15 reps per leg

SIDE LUNGES

- Stand with feet wider than shoulder-width apart.

- Bend your right knee, making sure not to extend it past your toes, while straightening your left leg.

- Keep your feet flat on the ground and facing forward.

- Complete the move by shifting your weight to the left side, bending your left knee and straightening your right leg.

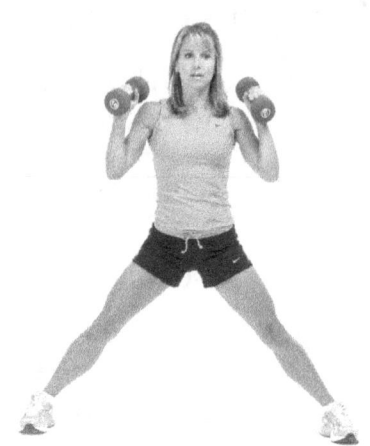

- Move back and forth, keeping as much of your weight back as possible as if you were sitting on a chair.

- Keep your back straight and shoulders back.

- Each time you lunge to each side, it counts as one rep.

- Make sure NOT to let your knee extend past your toes.

BEGINNER:
- 30 reps and build up to 50 reps.

ADVANCED:
- Add 5-20 pound dumbbells and complete 30 reps and then build up to 50 reps.

SQUATS

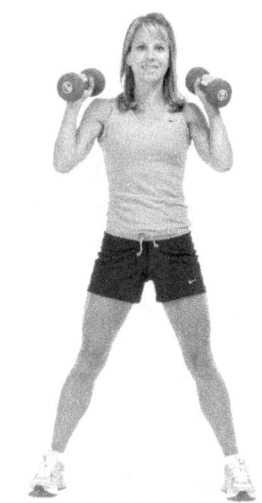

- Stand with feet shoulder-width apart.

- Lower your body down, bending the knees to a 90° angle.

- Make sure not to extend your knee past your toes.

- Keep your back straight, abs tight, and torso strong.

- Straighten your legs and squeeze your buttocks as you stand.

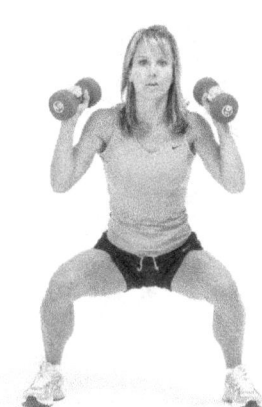

- Repeat.

BEGINNER:
- 10-30 reps.

ADVANCED:
- Add 5-20 pound dumbbells and complete 10-30 reps.

CALF RAISES

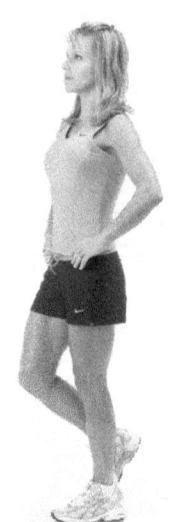

- Stand on your right leg, holding onto something for balance without putting your weight on it.

- Raise your body up onto the ball of your foot and then lower.

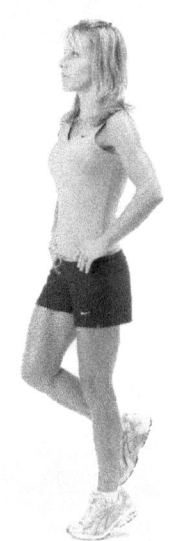

- Repeat.

- Complete a set and then change legs.

BEGINNER:
- Complete 10-15 reps per leg.

ADVANCED:
- Add 5-20 pound dumbbells and complete 10-30 reps per leg.

PELVIC BRIDGES

 • Lie on your back with legs bent and both feet flat on the floor, hip-width apart.

• Keep your arms on the floor by your sides.

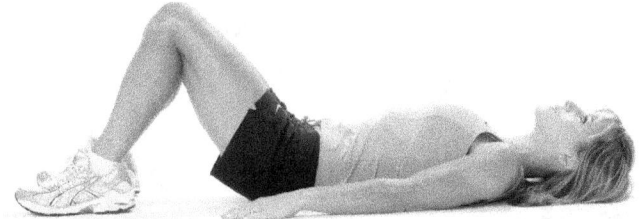

 • Keep your arms on the floor by your sides.

• Raise your hips up while tightening your buttocks and pressing down on your heels.

• Pulse up three times, and then lower to starting position, completing one rep.

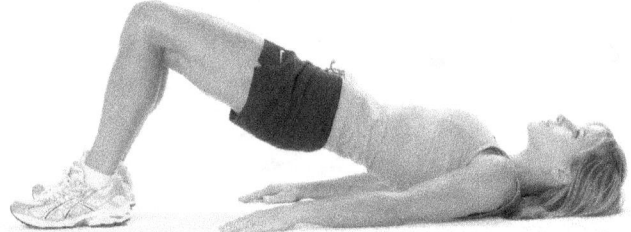

BEGINNER:
• 10-30 reps.

ADVANCED:
• Straighten your right knee using only your left leg for support as you complete the exercise.

• Complete 10-30 reps and then switch legs.

STEP-UPS

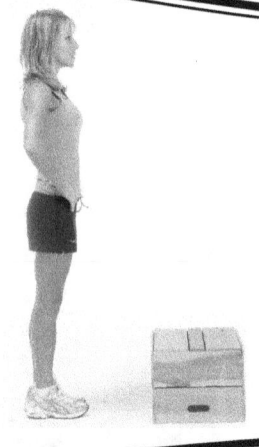

- Stand a few feet in front of a sturdy platform such as the hearth of a fire place, a bench, step, or workout platform.

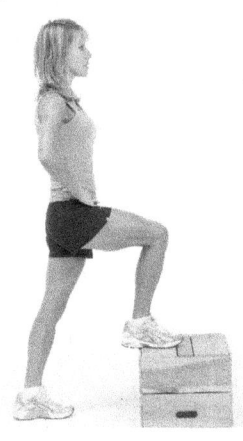

- Take a step up onto the top of the platform with your right leg and then bring your left leg up to meet it.

- Keep your back straight and head up. Immediately step back down with your left followed by the right.

NOTE:
The last leg to touch the platform is the first leg to step back down on to the floor.

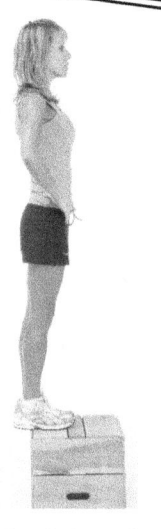

- Complete a set using the same leg to step up each time then switch to the other leg.

BEGINNER:
- 8-15 reps per leg.

ADVANCED:
- Add 5-15 pound dumbbells and complete 8-15 reps per leg.

UPPER BODY:

OVER-HEAD EXTENSIONS

- Stand with feet shoulder-width apart and knees slightly bent.

- Hold a 5 pound dumbbell in your left hand.

- Bend your left arm behind your head so your elbow points up to the ceiling.

- Support your left arm with your right hand just under your elbow, to ensure it stays in the proper position.

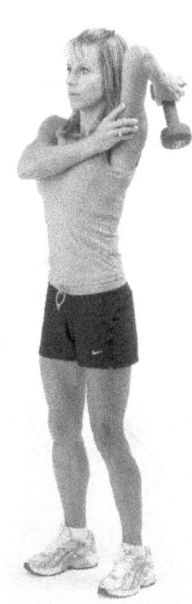

- Slowly straighten your upper arm while keeping your elbow stationary.

- Lower your upper arm back down.

- After completing a set, repeat using the right arm.

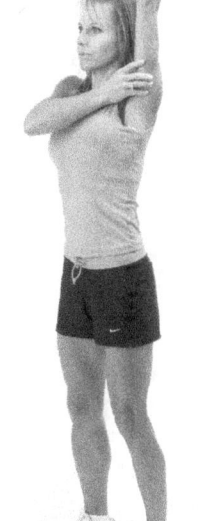

BEGINNER:
- 8-15 reps with a 5 pound dumbbell.

ADVANCED:
- Increase to a 10 pound weight and complete 8-15 reps

KICKBACKS

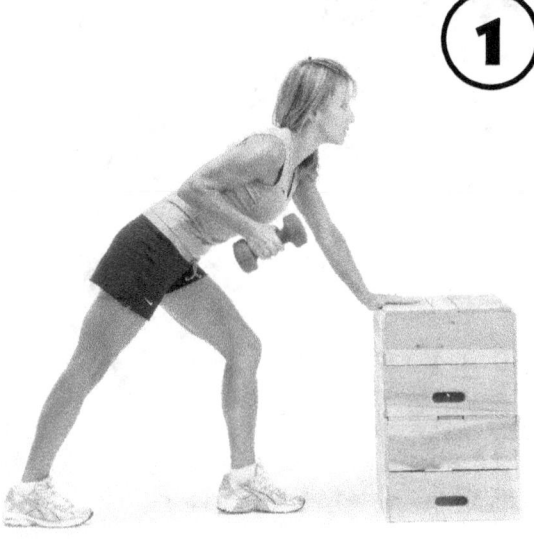

1 • Use a bench, table, or chair to support your body with your left arm.

• Step your left foot forward with knee slightly bent.

• Step back with your right foot for balance; keep back leg straight.

• Hold a dumbbell in your right hand; bend your elbow at a right angle, keeping your elbow pressed against your side.

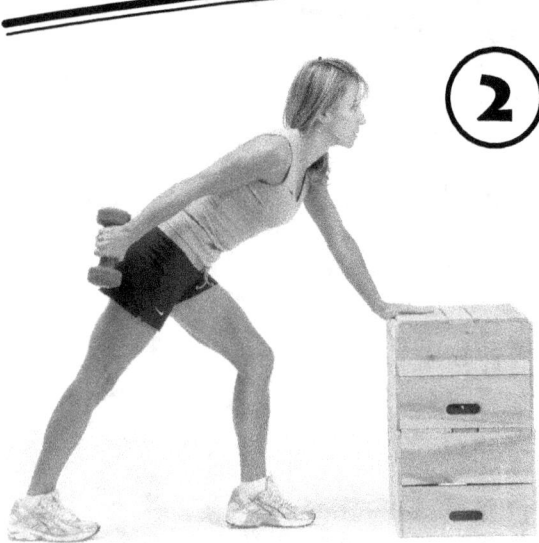

2 • With your palm facing your body, extend your arm back without moving your elbow or upper arm.

• Slowly return your arm to starting position.

• Complete a set then repeat with other arm.

BEGINNER:
• 8-12 reps with 5-10 pound weights.
ADVANCED:
• 10-20 reps with 10-20 pounds weights.

BICEP CURLS

1

- Stand with feet shoulder-width apart and knees slightly bent.

- Hold dumbbells at side and lift your right arm up, palms facing up.

- Keep your elbow tucked into your body and elbow stationary.

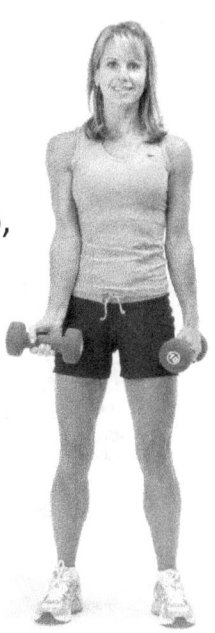

2

- Slowly lower and repeat with left arm.

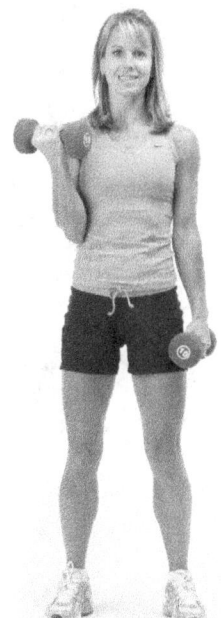

BEGINNER:
- 8-12 reps, per arm with 5-8 pound dumbbells.

ADVANCED:
- 8-12 reps, per arm with 10-15 pound dumbbells.

FRONT SHOULDER RAISES

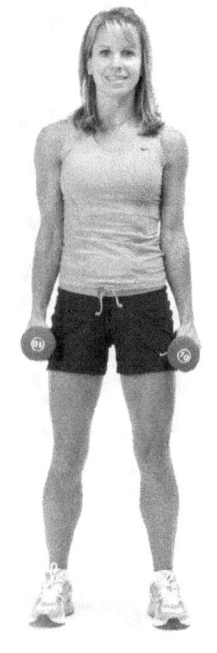

1

- Stand with feet shoulder-width apart and knees slightly bent.

- Hold dumbbells in each hand by your side with palms facing your body.

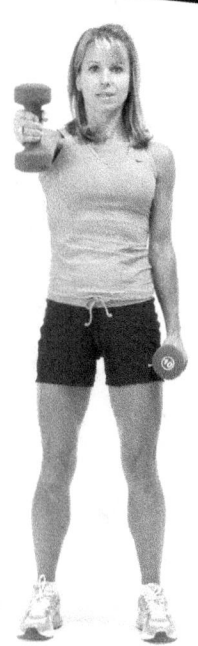

2

- Lift right arm to shoulder height in a slow motion.

- Keep your arm straight but not locked and slowly lower to your side.

- Repeat with your left arm.

BEGINNER:
- 8-12 reps, per arm with 5 pound weights.

ADVANCED:
- 8-12 reps, per arms with 8-10 pound weights.

BENCH DIPS

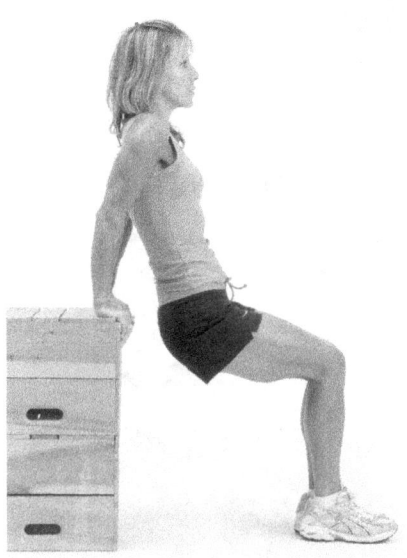

1

- With your back to a bench, chair or other platform, place your hands on the edge of the bench keeping your feet flat on the floor in front of you and knees at a 90° angle.

> MAKE SURE TO USE YOUR ARMS AND NOT YOUR LEGS, TO LIFT YOUR BODY UP AND DOWN.

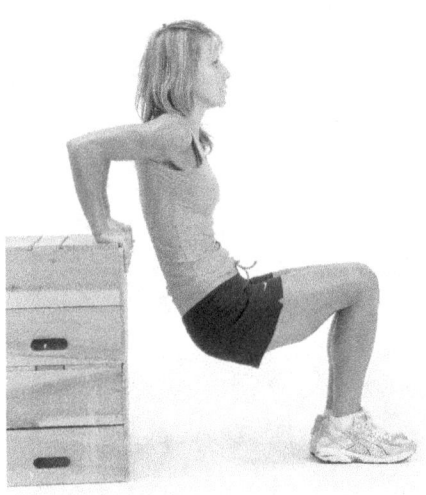

2

- Start with your arms straight and slowly bend your elbows to a 90° angle.

- Keep your elbows close to your body and pointing straight back.

- Slowly straighten your arms returning your body to the original position.

BEGINNER:
- 8-15 reps.

ADVANCED:
- Place a weight of 5-20 pounds on your upper thighs and complete a set of 8-25 reps.

ROTATOR CUFF EXCERSIZE
(SHOULDER)

- Stand with legs shoulder width apart.

- Hold a dumbbell in your right hand in front of you with arm at a right angle.

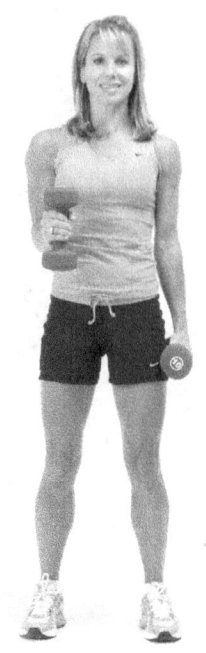

- Slowly rotate your arm to the right as far as you can then slowly return to the starting position.

- Complete a set then repeat with your left arm.

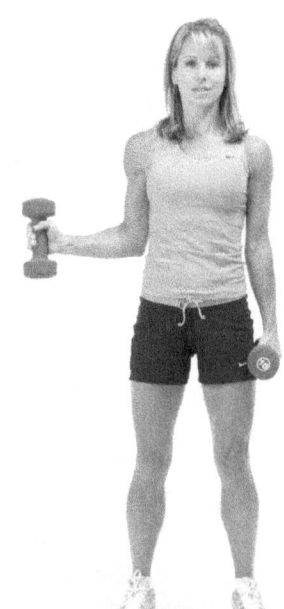

BEGINNER:
- 8-15 reps with a 5 pound dumbbell.

ADVANCED:
- 8-15 reps with a 10 pound dumbbell.

MODIFIED PUSH-UPS

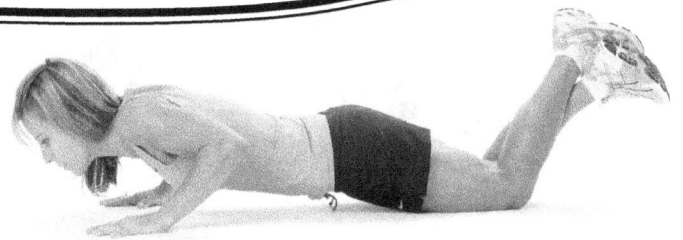

1
- Lie on the floor chest down with knees bent and feet crossed.
- Place hands under your shoulders on the floor.
- Keep your hands slightly more than shoulder-width apart and spread your fingers open to distribute your weight better, reducing the stress on your wrists.

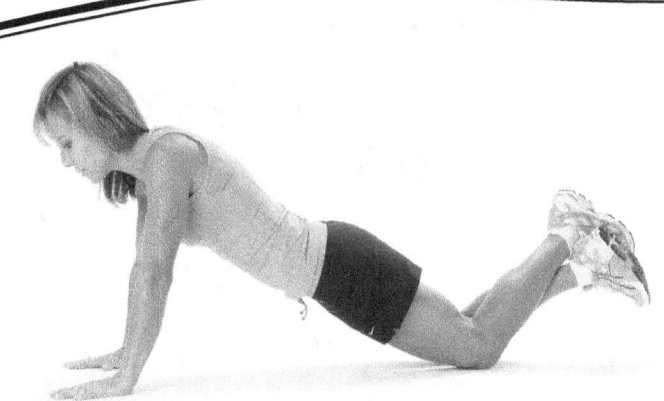

2
- Push up, exhaling as you straighten your arms.
- Keep your back straight and lower your body to the floor without touching it.
- Repeat.

BEGINNER:
- 8-12.

ADVANCED:
- 12-20 or advance to the traditional push-ups.

PUSH-UPS

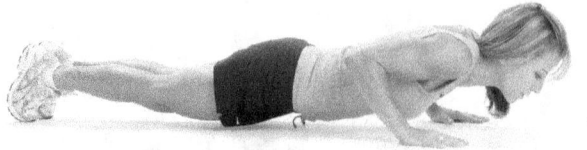

1 • Lie on the floor chest down, and place hands under your shoulders on the floor.

• Keep your hands slightly more than shoulder-width apart and spread your fingers open to distribute your weight better, reducing the stress on your wrists.

• Legs should be extended with your toes tucked under your feet.

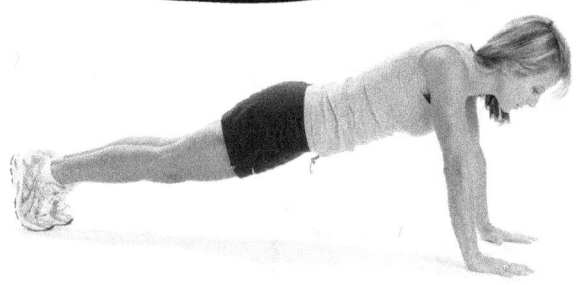

2 • Push up, exhaling as you straighten your arms.

• Your body should stay completely aligned. Inhale as you go back down.

• Get as close to the floor as you can without letting your body touch it.

• Complete as many as you are able without jeopardizing your form.

BEGINNER:
• 5-10.
ADVANCED:
• 10-20.

SINGLE-ARM ROWS

- Stand, legs staggered with left foot in front of the right.

- Slightly bend your left knee and keep your right leg straight.

- Make sure your knee doesn't extend past your toes.

- While holding a dumbbell in your right hand, use your left hand to support your upper body on the back of a chair or table.

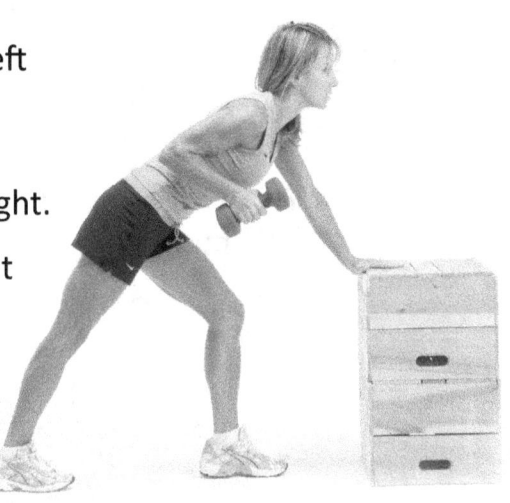

- Keeping your palm facing your body, lower your right hand down at an angle towards the chair.

- Draw dumbbell up to your rib cage while keeping your hips and shoulders squared.

- Slowly lower your arm back down.

- Complete a set then switch arms.

BEGINNER:
- 8-16 reps with 10 pound weights.

ADVANCED:
- 12-20 reps with 15-20 pound weights.

ABDOMINALS & CORE:

CRUNCHES

- Lie on the floor with knees bent.

- Place hands behind head for support, but don't use them to help push your body up as you do the exercise.

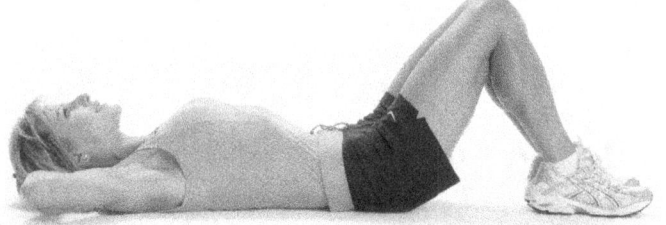

- Keeping your abs tight, lift your shoulders up towards the ceiling.

- Exhale as you lift up and inhale as you lower back to the floor.

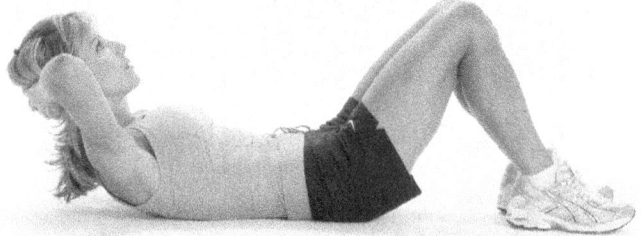

BEGINNER:
- Complete 8-25 reps.

ADVANCED:
- Complete the exercise as stated above but this time, cross your legs at the ankles and lift feet 2-3 inches off the floor with knees bent.

- Complete 8-25 reps.

REVERSE CRUNCHES

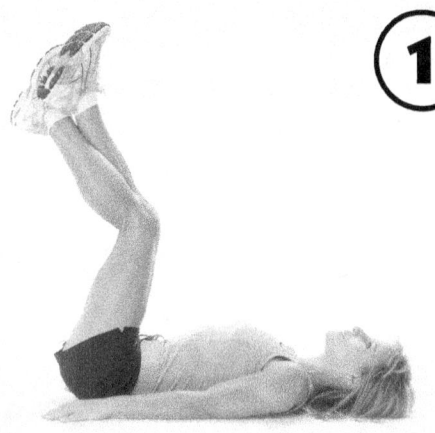

1

- Lie on the floor with your arms at your side.

- Raise your legs in the air so they are perpendicular to the floor.

- Keep knees slightly bent.

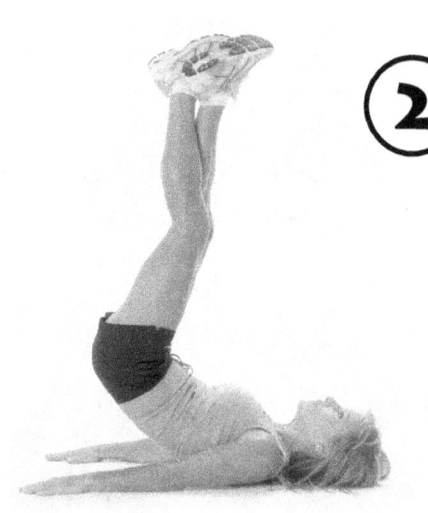

2

- Slowly lift hips up, keeping your shoulders on the floor.

- Lift as high as you can and hold before lowering them back onto the floor.

- Exhale as you lift.

BEGINNER:
- Complete 8-15 reps

ADVANCED:
- Extend your arms flat on the floor behind your head.

- Complete 8-15 reps.

DOUBLE CRUNCHES

1 • Lie on your back with hands behind your head, legs extended above the floor.

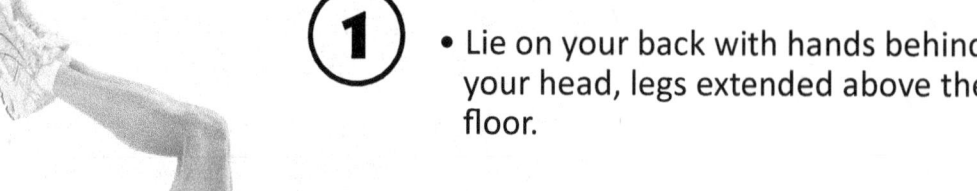

2 • Keeping abs contracted, curl your shoulders and bring your knees towards your chest and hold; lower back down without letting your feet or shoulders touch the floor.

• Exhale as your curl up.

BEGINNER:
• Complete 15 reps.
ADVANCED:
• Complete 16-30 reps.

BICYCLE CRUNCHES

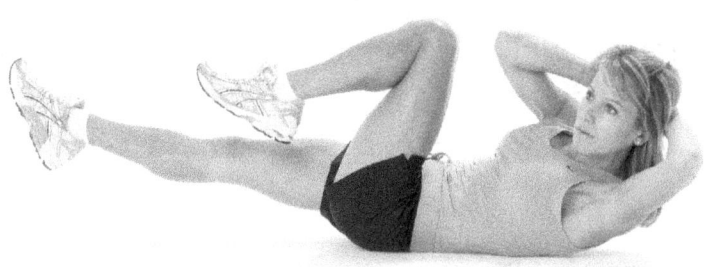

KEEP MOTION FROM YOUR SHOULDER AND NOT YOUR ELBOW.

1
- Lie on the floor with legs extended and hands behind your head.
- Bend your left knee toward chest and lift your right shoulder up and point elbow toward knee.

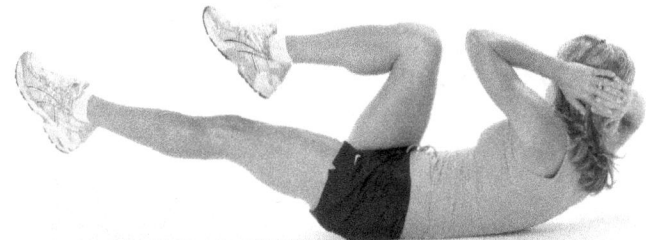

2
- Lower back to starting position and repeat on opposite side.
- Exhale as you lift up.

BEGINNER:
- Complete 15-30 reps.

ADVANCED:
- Hold each movement for 3 seconds before lowering back down.
- Complete 15-30 reps.

PLANKS

- Balance your body on your forearms with palms facing down.

- Straighten your body with toes on the floor so that your body is aligned and abs are contracted.

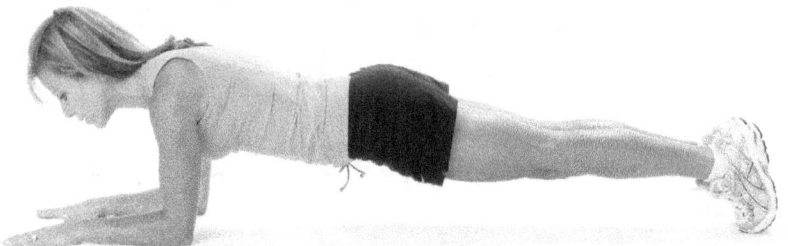

MAKE SURE TO KEEP YOUR BODY IN A STRAIGHT LINE

- Hold this position for 20-60 seconds.

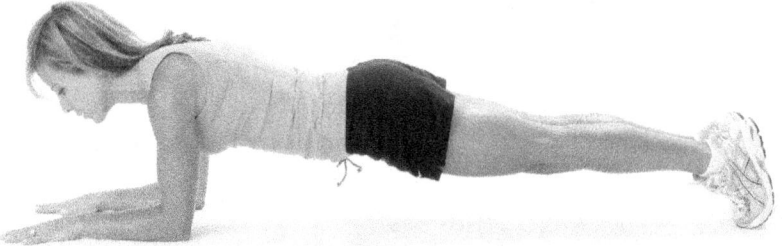

BEGINNER:
- Complete 1 set for 20-60 seconds.

ADVANCED:
- Complete 2-3 sets for 30-60 seconds.

STRETCHES:

LOWER BODY STRETCHES:

QUADRICEP STRETCH

- While standing, grasp the top of your left foot with your left hand and pull heel towards your buttocks. Push your foot against your hand until you feel the stretch in your thigh.

- Repeat with the left leg.

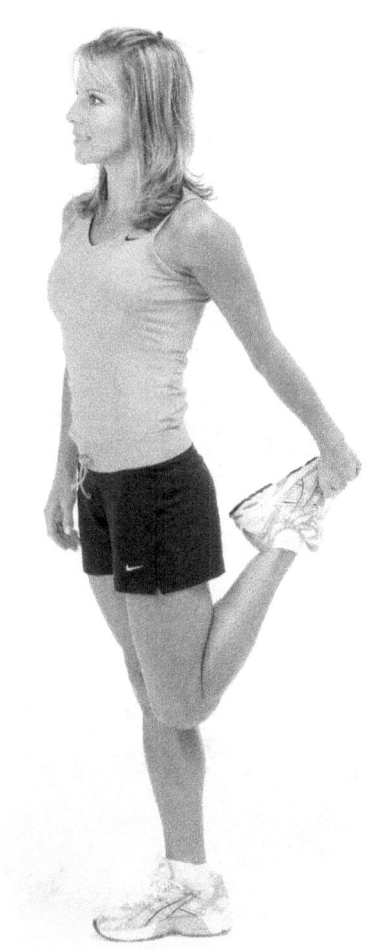

CALF STRETCH

- Standing in front of a wall, place your right heel as close as you can to the wall with toes pushed against wall.

- Left foot should be slightly back.

- Lean your body up against the wall; as you lean forward, the heel of your back foot should lift off the floor.

- Press down on the heel of your front foot to feel the stretch in your calf.

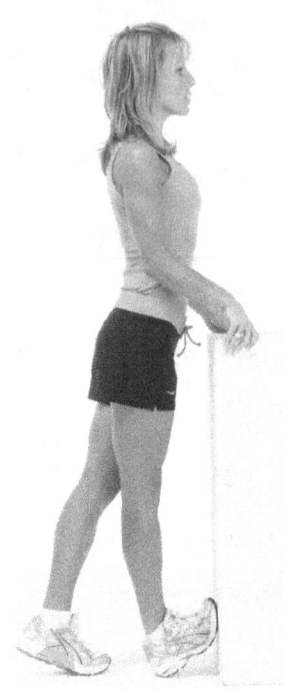

HAMSTRING STRETCH

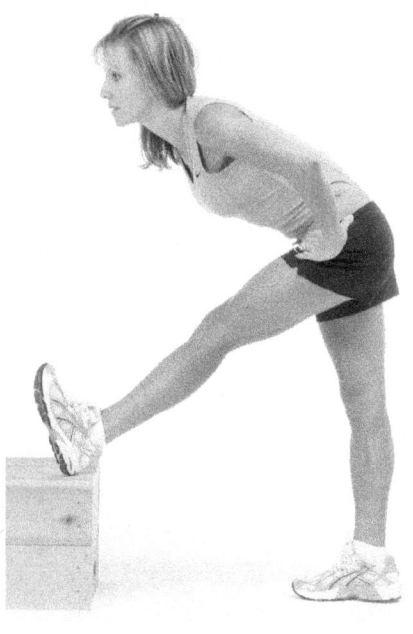

- Place the heel of your left foot on a chair, bench, or other sturdy elevated platform.

- Keeping elevated leg straight and hands on hips, lean forward until you feel the stretch in your hamstring.

SIDE LUNGE STRETCH

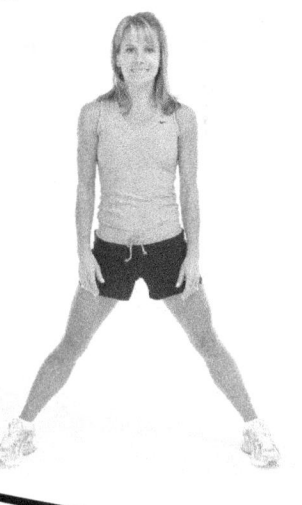

- Stand with feet wider than shoulder length apart.

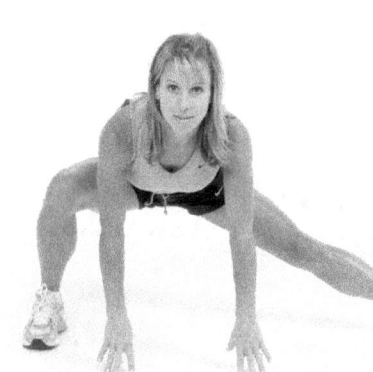

- Bend right leg as far as you can without extending knee past your toes; keep left leg straight as you bend and lean forward, resting hands on the ground in front of you.

- Hold for 15-30 seconds.

IF YOU DON'T FEEL THE STRETCH YOU NEED TO STAND WITH LEGS FARTHER APART.

- Next, turn your body to the right, rotating feet without moving them off the floor.

- Place your hands on both sides of your right foot and keep your back leg straight with front leg still bent at a 90 degree angle.

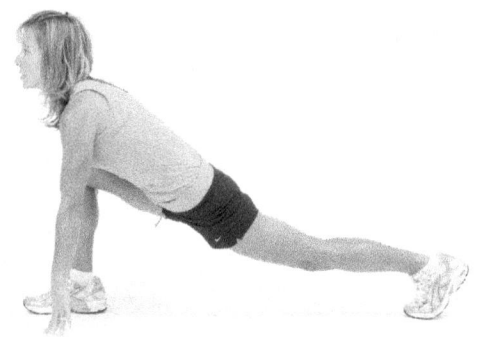

- Hold for 15-30 seconds.

- Repeat on other side.

UPPER BODY STRETCHES:

TRICEP SIDE STRETCH

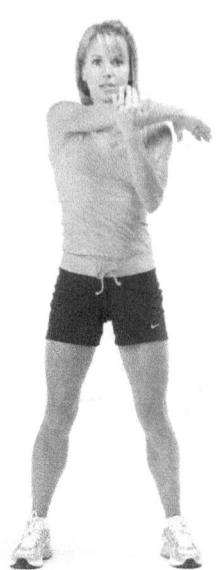

- Bring your right arm across your body and over your left shoulder.

- Hold your elbow with your left hand and gently push towards you while pushing out with your elbow until you feel the stretch in your tricep.

TRICEP OVERHEAD STRETCH

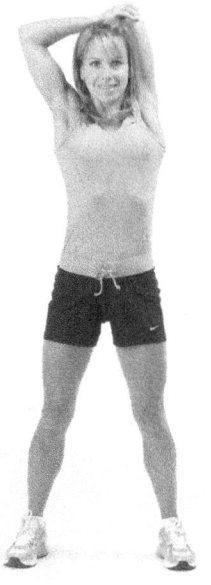

- Reach your left hand behind your head, grasp your elbow with your right hand and gently push downward while resisting with your elbow.

- Keep your back straight.

ELBOW CIRCLES:

SHOULDERS

- Stand with feet shoulder-width apart.

- Place hands on your shoulders with elbows pointing outward at shoulder level.

- Slowly make circles with elbows breathing out as you start the circle and breathing in as you finish it.

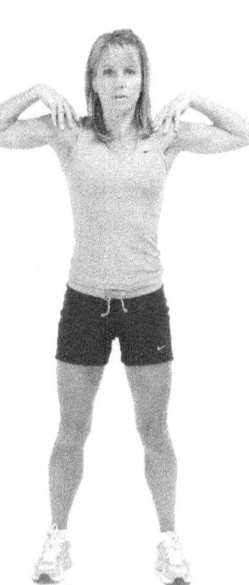

SHOULDER HUGS

- Hug yourself by grabbing hold of your back just under your shoulder blades.

- Try to pull blades away from each other with your hands.

- Lower your head forward to relieve neck tension while keeping shoulders down.

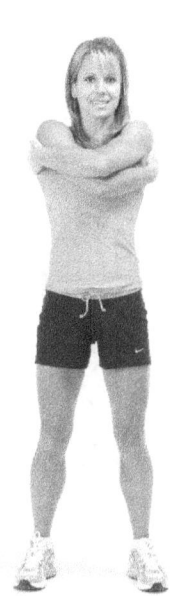

BICEP STRETCH

- Extend arms out in front of you with the palm of your right hand facing upward.

- With your left hand, grab the fingers of your right hand and push them back, resisting with your right arm.

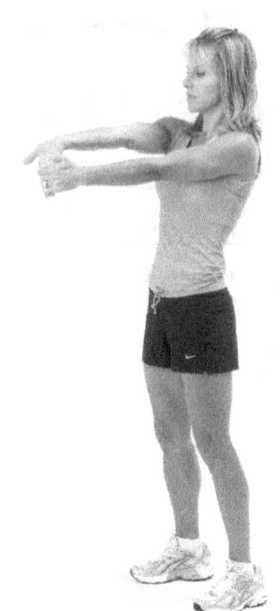

CHEST STRETCH

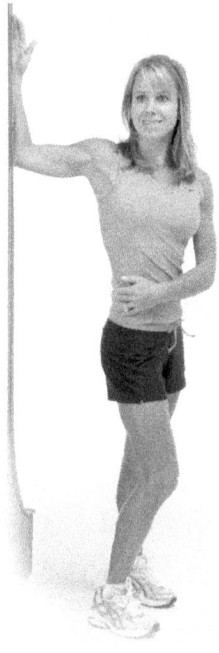

- Standing in a door frame, put your forearm on the frame so your arm is at a right angle.

- Step with your right leg slightly forward and rotate your hips to the left.

- Push with your forearm against the wall to feel the stretch in your chest.

- Repeat on the other side.

ABDOMINALS AND CORE BODY STRETCHES:

ABDOMINAL LATERAL STRETCH

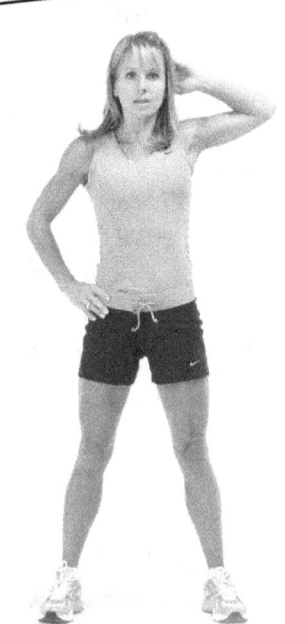

- Stand with feet slightly wider than your hips and slightly bend your knees.

- Place right hand on hip and left arm behind your head with elbow pointing outward.

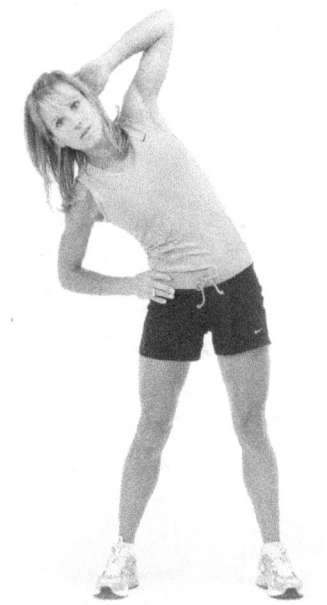

- Bend torso to the right keeping weight evenly distributed between both legs.

- Make sure to keep hips stationary.

- Bend until you feel a good stretch in your side abdominal muscles.

- Repeat with the other side.

KNEE HUG

- Lie on your back and bring both legs up to your chest; wrap your arms around them and hold.

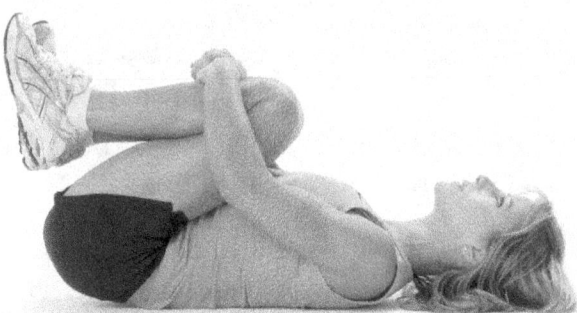

IF YOU HAVE KNEE PROBLEMS, HOLD YOUR LEGS TO YOUR BODY UNDER YOUR UPPER THIGH TO REDUCE THE STRESS ON THE KNEES.

LOWER BACK STRETCH

- Lie on your back and bring your left knee to your chest and hold with your hands; keep right leg straight and on the floor.

IF YOU HAVE KNEE PROBLEMS, HOLD YOUR LEGS TO YOUR BODY UNDER YOUR UPPER THIGH TO REDUCE THE STRESS ON THE KNEES.

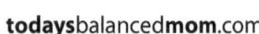

FLOOR TWIST

- Lie on the floor and bend knees.

- Twist your legs over your body and to the left, rotating at the hips.

- Place both arms to your right side, turning your head and upper body with your arms.

- Hold this position and repeat on the other side.

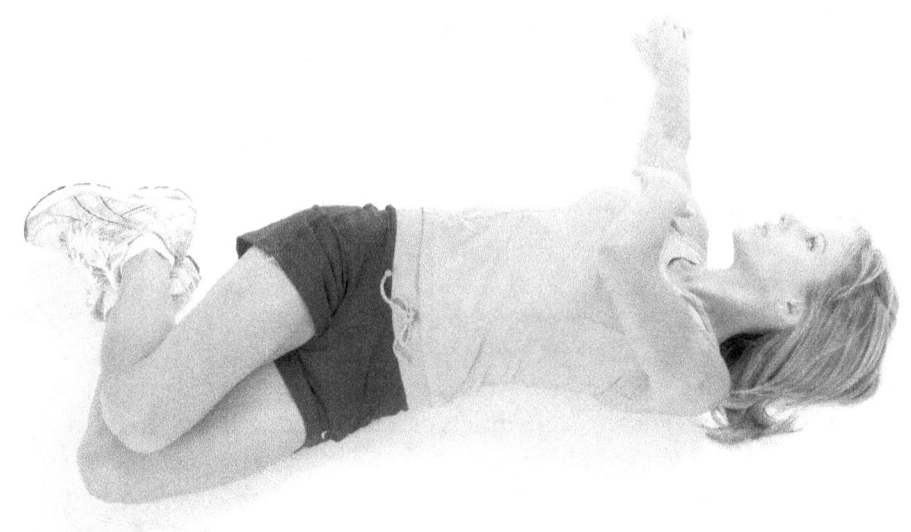

MAXIMIZE YOUR STRENGTH TRAINING:
FOLLOW THESE TIPS TO GET THE MOST OUT OF YOUR WORKOUT ROUTINE

• STRENGTH TRAIN 3 DAYS A WEEK WITH A DAY OF REST IN BETWEEN.

As you saw in the **28 Day Plan**, strength training should be performed three times a week with a day of rest in between each workout. This allows your muscles the time they need to recover. When you're lifting weights you're breaking down your muscle fibers and it's during the recovery period that you actually build your muscle back stronger than it was before.

• COMPLETE A FULL-BODY WORKOUT AT EACH STRENGTH TRAINING SESSION.

From the chart you can see that I recommend a full-body workout three days a week. Some people suggest targeting only certain groups of muscles and rotating each group throughout the week. I find this concept too time consuming because in order to work all your muscle groups, you'll have to spend more days working out. You can get the same results by completing a full-body workout in fewer days. You'll have to spend more time in each workout session to hit each muscle group completely, but overall you save in the time and days needed to strength train. Again, this is all about maximum results in minimal time!

• COMPLETE EACH SET TO FATIGUE.

Another strength training technique that gives you maximum results in minimal time is completing each set, or the number of repetitions of a particular exercise, to fatigue. This means performing one exercise to the point where you cannot finish the last repetition completely. Many people perform multiple sets with fewer repetitions and never reach the point of fatigue. Pushing to fatigue is a great time saver and you still get great results. The key here is to push yourself until you cannot easily complete the last rep of any particular exercise. You must work harder but you'll get the results you want in less time.

• ADJUST YOUR WEIGHT OR REPS AS NEEDED.

Whenever you can complete a set without reaching the point of fatigue, it's time to either increase the weight you're lifting or increase the amount of reps you're performing. If you're still trying to build muscle, you should add weight to the exercise. This is recommended for at least the first several months of your strength training routine. Once you see the results you're after, it's best to increase the reps that you perform so you keep working your muscles without getting bigger than you'd like. If you ever feel a certain muscle is larger than what you want, don't stop working out that muscle but instead, decrease the amount of weight you're using and increase the reps you complete.

• STRETCH EACH MUSCLE GROUP AFTER YOU WORK IT.

Another great way to maximize the look of your muscles and prevent injury is to stretch each muscle group after you work it. This can elongate the muscle instead of creating one small ball of muscle and gives you a great look of having muscle tone without looking too tight. Stretching each muscle group also helps prevent injury and promotes flexibility. It's easy to neglect this aspect of working out but you'll only be doing yourself a great disservice. You must allow time for appropriate stretching after each cardio activity and strength training exercise. Don't however, stretch out *before* you workout because your muscles will be cold and you could easily injure yourself. Wait until you have completed some cardio work and your muscles are warm, usually 5-10 minutes, if you like to stretch before you exercise. It's more important to stretch after your workout so make sure to allow about 5 minutes to give a good stretch to all of your muscle groups.

• WORK YOUR LOWER BODY FIRST, THEN UPPER BODY AND FINISH WITH ABDOMINALS.

It tends to be best to complete your lower body after your cardio, and then complete your upper body workout followed by your abdominal work. Your cardio gets the blood flowing to your leg muscles and it's beneficial to take advantage of that first before you move onto the other muscle groups. I prefer to end a strength training workout with abdominal moves because many are performed while lying down which decreases your heart rate.

• CREATE "MUSCLE CONFUSION".

Mix up the order you perform your exercises to create what is called muscle confusion. If you always workout with the same routine, your body anticipates this and your workout loses its effectiveness. Keep each move *within* the same muscle group but mix up the order you perform each move within that group. In other words, don't bounce around from an upper body move to several lower body moves, and then go back to another upper body move. Instead, change the order of the exercises *within* the same muscle group to take advantage of warm muscles. If you complete exercises that work several body parts at once, or compound exercises, this rule doesn't apply.

• WORK IN A CIRCUIT.

To maximize your workout, move from one strength training exercise to the next quickly. This keeps your heart rate elevated and allows you to complete your workout in a timely manner. Working out this way, known as circuit training, allows your strength training to take on the benefits of a cardio activity giving you double the benefits. You're essentially getting the benefits of both aerobic and anaerobic exercise in the same workout session. However, make sure you don't work the same muscle without giving it a break in between moves. You need to allow each muscle to rest before you work it again so alternate each specific muscle as you work through a circuit. Typically, you allow only 20 seconds at the most between each strength training move to get maximum results.

• DRINK WATER THROUGHOUT YOUR WORKOUT.

Your muscles need water to stay hydrated. Have water available throughout your workout routine and drink it liberally. Waiting until after you complete your workout is not as beneficial as drinking throughout your routine.

CHAPTER 7
SIMPLE TRICKS TO HELP YOU LOSE WEIGHT

If losing weight and keeping it off was easy, we wouldn't live in an overweight society. However, there are some simple tricks that can help you succeed in your weight loss effort. Make losing weight easier by incorporating some of the ideas below and you'll not only be able to stick to your **28 Day Plan**, but you'll be able to keep off the weight you lose for good!

• **If you don't buy it, you can't eat it.** It sounds like an obvious concept but a lot of people neglect to acknowledge the fact that if it's in your house you're going to be tempted by it. Don't buy foods that you know you can't resist. Even if ice cream or other off limits foods are on sale "buy one get one free" and it's hard to pass up the good bargain, you have to remember you might be saving a few dollars but you'll pay for it in pounds. For me, I'm easily tempted by high quality cheeses but don't care for the generic store brands. So to combat the temptation, I only buy the store brand cheese for my children so I don't have to test my will power. Why fight it? Just shop differently to ensure you don't have access to foods you'll regret eating later.

• **Buy snacks for your children that don't tempt you.** This concept is consistent with the one stated above. Buy food items for your children that you don't feel tempted by. I've never once been tempted by Goldfish, but my children love them. Consequently, that's the snack item that I purchase for them instead of baked chips which I know I'll end up eating. Know which foods tempt you and which ones you can resist, then adjust your grocery shopping to make eating right a lot easier.

• **Chew gum when you're making supper.** Most people tend to munch as they prepare supper and end up eating more fat and calories than they realize. If you pop in a piece of gum and chew it, you'll find it easier to resist sampling everything as you're preparing it.

• **Brush your teeth when you are tempted to eat what you shouldn't.** Food just doesn't taste as good right after you brush which makes saying no to temptation much easier. This little trick helps keep your eating in check; as a bonus it also improves your overall dental health.

• **Keep a healthy snack in your car or at your desk.** You know hunger is going to strike at certain times of the day. Having a healthy snack close at hand helps you to ward off that intense hunger that can make you overeat or choose convenient unhealthy foods. I always keep a can of reduced-sodium nuts in my car. Nuts are non-perishable, healthy, and loaded with protein that helps to keep my hunger in check. Have a stash of healthy snacks readily available so you can stay on track. Remember, this is not a green light to munch on your "emergency" snacks all day. You still need to write down what you're eating and keep your servings small.

• **When you feel hungry, drink water first.** Many times people mistake thirst for hunger. When you feel hunger kicking in yet you know you shouldn't be based on your food journal, try drinking a glass or two of water and let 20 minutes pass. By that time, either you'll have forgotten all about eating or your body got the water it was craving and you'll no longer feel hungry.

• **Drink a glass of almond milk, skim milk or soy milk when you come home hungry to take the edge off your hunger.** Drinking milk is a great way to help you feel full fast. If you walk in the door starving, drink a glass of milk before you do anything else to help you to stay in control of what you eat. My mom taught me this trick growing up. She would always drink a glass of skim-milk when she got home from work to curb her appetite and prevent her from binge eating. I love keeping a glass in the freezer to use for this purpose. It makes the milk ice cold and more satisfying to me.

• **Eat a large salad as an appetizer, or eat one as you prepare supper.** Salads are a great low-density food that keeps you satisfied. If you can eat one as your late afternoon snack you'll see a noticeable reduction in you hunger level come supper time. Eating a salad before your meal will help you consume fewer calories during your main course. Salads are low in calories, rich in nutrients and give you a feeling of fullness. Never use regular dressings to avoid consuming unnecessary fat, and watch for calories that can be found in the form of croutons, cheeses, etc..

• **Serve two vegetables with your meals instead of one.** We all know the great health benefits of vegetables so why limit ourselves to just one per meal? You really have to eat two servings of vegetables per meal in order to get the recommended daily intake every day. Vegetables fill you up with minimal calories and offer great health benefits so why not put two on your plate instead of one?

• **Add vegetables to your sandwiches to make them more filling and healthy.** If you add lettuce, tomatoes, sliced cucumbers, alfalfa sprouts, and red onions to your sandwich, not only have you added extra important vitamins and nutrients to your meal, but you'll feel fuller and more satisfied by only adding a few extra calories.

• **Prep vegetables and fruit to make for easy snacks.** Having healthy options ready to eat will make grabbing a quick snack not only healthy but easy. It also makes it easier to choose some that work with your diet instead of opting for other unhealthy and fattening choices you might be tempted by. When you get home from the store, wash and cut up some fruits and vegetables so they're ready to eat. You can even save time by having your children wash or cut, while you put away the rest of the groceries. Even the youngest of children can use a plastic lettuce knife to chop lettuce making putting together a salad that much easier. Try letting them use a salad spinner and you'll have an entertained child for hours and the driest washed lettuce in town!

• **Have vegetables out to snack on while you prepare supper.** You and your family will munch on whatever you have set out while waiting for supper time. Everyone's hungry and wants what's easy and available. If you put out some carrots and celery with fat-free or low-fat dressing, that's what they'll eat. This is a great way to help you stay on track and make sure your family is eating healthy at the same time without spoiling supper.

• **When you get the urge to munch, get active!** If you feel an eating binge coming on, do something physical. You can do a set of sit-ups, shoot hoops with your kids, take everyone for a quick bike ride or walk, or just horseplay with your children. It'll help get your mind off food, get your heart pumping and your metabolism revved up. I used this trick to help me get back into shape after giving birth – five times! Every time I felt like eating but knew I shouldn't, I dropped to the floor and did sit-ups. It was a double bonus because not only did it take my focus off food, but it also helped me get my abdominal muscles back into shape after childbirth. I also found it effective to just go outside whenever the temptation to eat set in.

• **After supper, close off the kitchen and stay out!** Lingering in the kitchen makes it harder to not think about food, and thinking about food usually leads to eating. Once the kitchen is cleaned for the night, turn off the lights and stay out.

• **Use spices to jazz up your food instead of salt or fat.** If you use the right spices and herbs you can increase the flavor of foods without adding fat or salt. You'll also get the added health benefit of the spices and herbs to increase the nutritional value of your meal. If you can, it's always best to use fresh instead of dried herbs and spices because of their higher nutritional value and enhanced flavor.

• **Keep foods out of sight that you shouldn't eat.** If you have foods in your house that are off limits to you, keep them out of sight. Don't test your will power by having a cookie jar filled with delicious treats on your counter that will tempt you every time you see it. Keep foods that tempt you out of sight and in a place that's difficult to get to. If you must have treats in your house, put them on the top shelf in your pantry or in a spare refrigerator so you have to work to get to them. Those extra steps or the energy of having to grab a stool to reach something, might require just enough effort to discourage you from indulging. It also gives you a few extra moments to think about what you're about to eat and whether it's worth it as compared to foods within easy reach that can be mindlessly eaten.

• **Keep a bowl of fresh fruit on your kitchen counter.** Apply the concept mentioned above by keeping *healthy* food available such as having a bowl of fruit on the counter. You're much more likely to eat fresh fruit if it's easily available and not lost in the bottom of your vegetable keeper. This helps to build healthy eating habits for your children too because the odds are higher that they'll eat more fruit instead of other less healthy snacks that are logistically more difficult to obtain. Everyone wants what's easiest so make eating healthy as easy as possible.

• **When you get the urge to eat something sweet, skip the chocolate and eat fresh fruit or yogurt.** We all get a sweet tooth now and then; it's what we do with it that makes the difference from a diet fumble or a diet success. Fruit is truly nature's candy and should be treated as such. If you crave something sweet, grab some watermelon or strawberries. You'll be surprised how satisfying it can be, especially once your taste buds have adjusted to your new way of healthy eating.

• **Sprinkle cayenne pepper on your foods to boost your metabolism.** Add a little cayenne pepper to your favorite dishes to give it some kick and to help rev your metabolism. Spicy foods such as jalapeño peppers work well for this and offer great health benefits because they're packed with vitamins and nutrients.

• **Use smaller plates and bowl for your meals.** If you use smaller serving dishes for your meals, you'll trick your brain into thinking you're eating *more* than if you use a bigger dish that makes your serving size look modest. It's proven people feel more satisfied when they eat a meal from a salad plate that looks full, versus a meal from a regular dinner plate that looks scarce.

CHAPTER 8
COMMON QUESTIONS AND ANSWERS ABOUT DIET AND FITNESS

How long will it take for me to see results from the 28 Day Plan?
You should start losing weight within the first week or two. You'll also feel an improvement in your energy level and overall health. It will take several weeks to see the results of your strength training but you'll feel the benefits and its positive effects on your weight loss effort quickly.

I just had a baby and am nursing. Is this eating plan safe for me?
Congratulations on making the choice to nurse your baby! Nursing your baby is the best gift you can give to your child. Nursing is also a benefit to you because it helps you return to your pre-pregnancy weight faster due to the extra calories you burn to produce milk. It's also a great way to get your uterus back to its original size. Eating healthy is very important when you nurse because of the demands on your body and because you want your baby to receive as many vitamins and nutrients through your milk as possible. This eating plan is an excellent way for you to get back to your pre-pregnancy weight because it incorporates eating pure foods and encourages exercise which is good for the both of you. Limiting all the "bad" you eat such as artificial additives and preservatives, is also very important because it's transferred to your baby through your milk.

To compensate for the extra calories needed to produce adequate milk, you do need to add to the total number of calories allowed per day to lose weight safely. On average, a nursing mother should consume an additional 300-500 calories per day. You should NEVER go below 1800 calories. You should also wait about six weeks before cutting calories too much to allow your milk supply to get established and to help your body recover from childbirth. If you're like me, this won't be a problem because you'll be starving during this time period and cutting calories will be difficult. Don't worry though, you will be losing weight during this time period naturally. You can begin eating the foods on the **28 Day Plan**, just allow more calories and then gradually decrease the amount you consume as your milk stabilizes and your body recovers from giving birth. You can also gradually start exercising after childbirth to help get your body back into shape. Always consult your obstetrician first, but most moms who deliver vaginally can begin brisk walking 1-2 weeks after delivery. Listen to your body and increase your cardio workout as you and your doctor see fit. I don't recommend running or intense strength training until after your post-delivery check-up. There are some basic exercises you can do to get your muscles going again. Just start off easy and work your way into the recommended routine. (One exercise you *can* do immediately after delivery is the Kegel exercise. Kegels are important to getting your vaginal muscles back to where they should be and the earlier you start them, the better. Your doctor can give you information on how to do these properly.)

When trying to lose weight while nursing, keep in mind that your body's health will suffer if you restrict calories too much. In order to provide your baby with the nutrients he needs, vitamins and minerals will be stripped from your body if they're not provided in the food you consume. This eating plan is a perfect way for you to accomplish losing weight and provide you and your baby with the nutrients you *both* need. You just have to make sure you're consuming the necessary calories to ensure adequate milk supply by losing weight gradually. You also don't want to lose weight too quickly because when you lose weight too fast, your body burns extra fat which releases toxins that are stored in your fat tissues contaminating your milk. Losing two pounds per week is considered a safe amount for nursing moms.

Is it OK to drink diet soft drinks since they have zero calories?

NO! You can save the diet drinks for an occasional indulgence but they shouldn't be a regular part of your diet. Even though they don't contain any calories, they still play a negative part in your overall health and diet effort. There are health risks involved with artificial sweeteners and some studies have shown that there's an actual *increase* in appetite when zero calories sweeteners are consumed. Another negative is that most sweeteners are up to 700 times sweeter than table sugar. Consuming this high concentration of sweetness can distort our natural taste for the sweetness of foods. This sabotages your diet effort because it'll take extremely sugary foods to satisfy your sweet tooth and natural foods won't be as satisfying as they would otherwise.

I've always avoided nuts because they're so high in fat and calories. Why do you have them a part of the 28 Day Plan?

Nuts are high in fat but they're the good fats including monounsaturated, polyunsaturated and omega-3 fats which help keep hunger at bay and are very heart healthy. Even with their high fat and calories, nuts can actually help you *lose* weight. A study was conducted that had two groups consume the same amount of calories; one group was allowed to eat 3 ounces of almonds and the second group wasn't. After twenty-four months the group that consumed the almonds lost 62% more weight, had a 50% greater reduction in fat mass and a 50% greater reduction in waist circumference. As this study shows, nuts can be a great part of your overall weight loss effort and overall improvement of your health. I've eaten more nuts in the past three years than I have in my entire life and I weigh what I did in middle school. Keep a can of low-salt or unsalted nuts handy to help you in your diet success. Your best choices are walnuts, almonds, and Brazilian nuts. (This study was taken from the *International Journal of Obesity* November 2003 issue.)

With my hectic mornings, finding time to eat breakfast is very difficult for me. Can I lose the weight I want and still skip this meal?

You could probably still lose weight without incorporating breakfast into your day but it would be much harder and take a lot longer. Your general health may also suffer. Breakfast *is* the most important meal of the day and every effort should be made to make it a part of your diet. You don't have to sit down to a full meal to reap the benefits however. Keep a can of nuts or a protein bar in your bathroom to eat while you're getting ready and breakfast is served! No one is too busy to do that. It's worth making time for breakfast to get your metabolism working again after a night of fasting. Eating breakfast will also help you feel fuller throughout the day reducing the total amount of calories you eat.

To reduce my total sodium intake, will cutting out the salt I add to foods be enough to make a difference?

No, salt hides in many places you might never expect. While cutting out table salt will reduce your total intake, you're more than likely still consuming more sodium than you should. One morning I awoke feeling like I had eaten a salt stick and couldn't understand why since I'd only eaten a salad with grilled chicken strips for supper. I finally discovered that the Italian fat-free salad dressing I used as a marinade for the chicken contained more salt than *two* servings of salted pretzels. I would have never guessed there was that much salt in salad dressings. Many processed foods, sauces and marinades have very high salt content so make sure to read the labels. Consuming too much salt is going to make you retain unnecessary water, leave you bloated and increase your risk of health problems. Purchase reduced-sodium products as often as you can to help reduce your salt intake. When you eat out you'll definitely consume more salt than you would by eating at home. In fact, many meals contain more than *half* of the maximum daily recommended salt intake. The FDA has suggested the maximum sodium intake for a healthy diet to be about 2,400 mg. Strive to keep your sodium intake much less than this number, and your health will improve as well as your appearance because you won't be retaining as much water.

It's also important to avoid or curtail your consumption of processed foods including deli meats, chips, crackers, snack items, and fast foods. These foods contain very high levels of sodium. Even foods that you might think would be a healthy option like a Chargrilled Chicken Sandwich from Chik-fil-A, contains 1300 mg of sodium. That's 54% of the maximum suggested intake in one sandwich.

What can I do if I don't like fruits and vegetables?

It's time for you to develop a liking for them not only for your diet effort but for your overall health. Continue to try different fruits and vegetables while reminding yourself of their importance to your body and you should eventually develop a taste for them. It's also important for your children to see you eat and enjoy fruits and vegetables because their eating habits will emulate yours. Make the effort to eat more fruits and vegetables and before you know it, you'll enjoy their flavor and the benefits they have on your weight loss effort and health in general.

Should I always purchase fresh fruits and vegetables or can I buy them frozen or canned?

Fruits and vegetables that are frozen can be just as good for you as buying them fresh. They're usually flash frozen which preserves their vitamins, nutrients and flavor. In fact, frozen can sometimes be even healthier than fresh because by the time produce gets to your table it could have been picked weeks ago. This is a negative because as soon as produce is picked it begins to lose its nutrients and flavor. Usually you can look at the produce and tell if it's been on the shelf too long because it looks and feels limp or is browning. I like to buy fresh produce that's in season, and buy frozen when an item is out of season. Another benefit of buying frozen fruits and vegetables is you always have something on hand to help make a healthy meal at a moment's notice.

Try to avoid canned fruits and vegetables if possible. They tend to be high in sodium and the fruits are usually packed in syrup. Canned tomatoes and tomato products are usually fine to purchase. In fact, canned tomatoes contain more lycopene which protects against heart disease and some cancers than fresh tomatoes. If you must purchase canned vegetables, choose the low-sodium varieties, or rinse the vegetables to reduce the amount of salt they contain. To prevent contamination from the can's liner, NEVER store food in an open can in the refrigerator. Always transfer the food to another storage container - preferably glass.

I'm having a hard time giving up dessert. What can I do to satisfy my sweet tooth?

Once your taste buds adjust to your new way of eating, satisfying your sweet tooth can be accomplished by eating fresh fruits such as watermelon, strawberries or pineapple. Until then, try low-fat yogurt or even frozen low-fat yogurt, just make sure you limit your portions and frequency. A piece of dark chocolate can end your craving and is actually very good for you. I love adding frozen blueberries to my morning cereal for a sweet treat and an extra boost of vitamins and nutrients. A sweet fix doesn't have to come in the form of chocolate cake or a candy bar. Even hot cocoa with skim milk can calm your sweet tooth without doing much damage to your diet efforts. While you're using the **28 Day Plan** avoiding desserts will help you reach your goal much faster. Once your weight is where you want it to be, indulging once in a while is fine. Just keep the portions small and infrequent. Also, try to cut calories from other foods to help make up for the extra ones consumed from your dessert.

The holidays are coming up and I'm worried I won't be able to stick to my eating plan. What can I do to stay on track?

It's not uncommon to put on a few pounds during the holiday season, much less expect to lose weight. In fact, it's more uncommon NOT to gain weight during this festive time of year. Great food, delicious desserts, holiday libations – the temptations are everywhere. Add into the equation that you have less time and energy to squeeze in a workout and you have a formula for a diet disaster. It's almost impossible to avoid all the delicious foods but you can be smart and minimize the damage the holiday season can have on your weight loss effort. Follow these simple tips to help stay on track:

1. Reduce your portion size of foods that are high in calories and fat. If you can't resist that homemade macaroni and cheese on Thanksgiving Day, serve yourself only *half* of what you'd normally eat. It's fun to sample all the wonderful foods but you don't have to eat a full serving of each. You can still allow yourself the pleasure of eating some of your favorite holiday foods, just keep the portions small.

2. Don't indulge in the leftovers. Many times the extra calories and fat you consume during the holidays come not from the big family dinner itself, but the leftovers you eat the days after. It makes it easier if you're eating Thanksgiving or Christmas dinner at another family member's house since the leftovers stay there. If you take a dish to share you can leave your remaining food with the hostess so you're not tempted by it at home. If the meal is at your house, send home leftovers with your guests for them to enjoy and to get them out of your house. Freezing leftovers is another great way to get the food out of sight and to have an easy meal or side dish for your family later on.

3. Keep candies and desserts out of sight. As stated before, don't test your will power by having a cookie jar filled with delicious treats on your counter that will tempt you every time you see it. Keep foods that tempt you out of sight and in a place that's difficult to get to. Put treats on the top shelf in your pantry or in a spare refrigerator so you have to work to get to it. Those extra steps or the energy of having to grab a stool to reach something might require just enough effort to discourage you to indulge. This will also gives you a few extra moments to think about what you're about to eat and whether it's worth it versus if the food is within easy reach and can be mindlessly eaten.

4. Indulge only in the foods that are really worth it. Why eat the fat and calories of a slice of pecan pie if you don't absolutely love it? Be aware of what you're putting in your mouth and ask yourself if you'll enjoy it enough to be willing to work off the fat and calories. Consider this; a slice of pecan pie can easily contain over 500 calories and 27 grams of fat. You'd have to run 5-6 miles to burn off that one slice of pie. If you're a huge pecan pie fan it might be worth it to you. But if you can take it or leave it, I'd leave it.

5. Make an effort to stick to your exercise routine. To burn off the extra calories you'll be consuming, you need to make sure you fit exercise into your schedule. Try to add any additional exercise to your routine if possible. You might have to get creative to find the time to workout with all the added demands around the holidays, but it's worth it. You'll not only keep the weight off but your sanity will benefit. Exercise is a great stress reliever and will help you better handle all that you have to do. When your kids are out of school, incorporate your workouts so they can participate with you. Use a baby jogger to go for a power walk, run while they ride bikes, rent an exercise DVD that they can participate in, etc. Get creative and make it happen! You'll be glad you did.

6. Remember, every calorie counts! The mentality of most people is that if they've already blown their diet, they might as well go all out and eat whatever they want. Don't fall into this trap. Every calorie you put into your mouth has to be burned off. If you over did it on one meal, you can make up for it by adding in an extra workout, but if you over do it a second time you'll have to work *twice* as hard to burn off the calories. Your body doesn't care what your justifications are for eating what you do, it only knows that if the calories aren't burned off, it has to store them which results in weight gain.

These **6 simple tips** can help prevent gaining holiday pounds by balancing the temptations with smart choices. Doing this will allow you to enjoy the holiday fare while also helping you look *and* feel better when the season's over. What a great way to start the New Year!

Because of work, I tend to eat out for lunch every day and often entertain clients over dinner. Can I still reach my goals?

Eating out frequently makes sticking to your **28 Day Plan** and maintaining weight loss much more difficult. Most meals contain about 60% more calories than that same dish if you prepared it at home. If you can't avoid eating out by packing a lunch for work, you need to be very careful when ordering. Knowledge is your best weapon against the temptations of restaurant foods. Some restaurants provide a nutritional information guide or list the information on the menu. For those that don't, there are some great websites that will give you the nutritional information for a lot of the country's popular restaurants. Check out food establishments that you frequent and look up the calories and fat of their menu selection. This will allow you to know what you're about to eat before you order and you'll be able to record the information in your food journal to keep you within your daily caloric allotment. If you can't find what the nutritional value of a particular restaurant's offerings are, use the guide below to help you make the wisest choices:

• *Pick restaurants that have a salad bar so you can control exactly what you eat. Avoid fatty dressing, croutons, full-fat cheeses, and the mayonnaise salads that are often found in salad bars.*

• *If a salad bar isn't available, choosing a mixed green salad is always your best choice. If they don't have a fat-free or low-fat dressing, ask for vinegar and olive-oil or just squeeze a fresh lemon over your salad. If you order a low-fat dressing ask that it come on the side so you can control how much of it you eat.*

• *Avoid all pasta entrees.*

• *Ask that the bread that often comes with a meal not be brought to the table.*

• *Substitute steamed vegetables or a side salad for the baked potato or rice.*

• *Order water, unsweetened tea, or coffee to save on calories. When ordering tea, I always ask my server to mix half unsweetened with half sweetened tea. This allows me to get a glass of iced tea with a little sweetness but without **all** the extra calories. Ideally the tea should be unsweetened but again, due to my Southern roots I still have to have a little sugar in there.*

• *Try to order entrees that include skinless chicken breasts, seafood (grilled or broiled), wild game or beans. If you prefer to order meat, look for filets, tenderloin, flank steak, top sirloin or top rounds.*

• *Never, never, order anything fried!*

• *Avoid dishes that contain words such as cream sauce, butter sauce, Alfredo, bisque, or white sauce. Opt instead for dishes that use a tomato base or a red sauce.*

• *If the menu doesn't give good detail, ask how a dish is prepared and if necessary, find out if it can be altered into a low-fat version.*

• *Split an entrée with a friend or spouse.*

• When you receive your meal, discretely divide it in half and only eat one of the portions. Save the other half to take home.

• Ask that the kitchen box up half the meal before they bring it to the table. This is a guaranteed way to prevent overeating.

• Drink a glass of water before the meal is served to help you feel fuller and to aid in digestion.

• Order an appetizer as your meal. This can give you a smaller portion but be careful of what your order as sometimes it's hard to find a healthy appetizer.

• Order a tomato, bean or broth based soup. Soup will help you fill up and when eaten with a salad, it can be a very satisfying meal without sabotaging your diet. Avoid cream-based soups due to their high fat and calorie content.

• Have your plate removed as soon as you start to feel full so you're not tempted to continue eating. You can even ask that it be removed right before a sense of fullness occurs because as time passes, you'll feel fuller since it takes time for your brain to tell your stomach that you're no longer hungry.

• Avoid all-you-can-eat buffets.

• If you order a sandwich, ask for mustard instead of mayonnaise.

• Don't eat the bun or bread on a sandwich. If you want to eat some bread, order whole wheat and don't eat the top slice to cut back on calories and carbohydrates. Use a fork and knife to eat the sandwich gracefully and prevent having a mess on your hands - literally.

You recommend using olive oil. Which kind is the best to purchase?

Olive oil has an impressive list of benefits. It should always be your first choice when using oil. The best olive oil is first cold-pressed extra virgin. It's derived from the first pressing of olives and has the most antioxidant benefits and a delicate flavor. Make sure to store your olive oil in a cool, dark place and use it within a year to get the most health benefit and flavor. Olive oils that come in dark bottles are an even better choice because the dark color of the glass protects it from the light.

In the strength training program, you recommend one set of a certain move when I've always read to complete several sets in a workout. Why?

Busy moms like us know that getting maximum results in minimal time is important in everything we do. I've found through research and personal experience that great results can be attained by only completing one set of an exercise *if* it's completed to fatigue. This technique can cut your workout time almost in half and can give you the same, if not better results. Working to fatigue requires that you push yourself so the last rep is very difficult, if not impossible to complete.

Is there a better time of the day to workout?

The morning time is the preferred workout time for several reasons. First of all, you get it done and don't have the excuses or distractions that can come up during your day to keep you from exercising. Secondly, studies have shown that your metabolism will be positively affected by your morning workout and you'll burn more calories throughout the day. Lastly, you'll feel great all day because you know you've accomplished something for yourself and are doing what it takes to reach your goal. Of course if it doesn't fit into your schedule to work out in the morning, working out anytime is a great time. Your lunch break might be when you can fit in a run or gym visit, or immediately after work. What ever you need to do, just fit a workout in somehow.

I'm so pushed for time during my workout, is it really necessary for me to spend the time stretching out?

Yes! Stretching helps to prevent injury, promotes flexibility and lengthens the muscle you're working out to create a nice toned lean look. For the extra time it takes to stretch, it's well worth it.

Is it possible to target and burn fat from a specific area?

No. However you burn calories, whether through a cardio workout or lifting weights, fat cells will shrink all over your body and not in one specific area. If you want a certain part of your body to look better, lifting weights to target that area will help to tone the muscle underneath the fat. Once you get the fat off, you'll reap the rewards with a beautifully toned muscle that's been waiting to show itself off!

I see people in the gym complete their weight training in fast, quick motions. Is that right?

Most of the time the answer to that question is no. Your body gets better results by completing a rep in a slow and controlled movement. It challenges your muscles more and will give you better results. Keep in mind that the second part of a move is just as important as the first part and should be controlled and slow. For example, when doing a bicep curl lowering your forearm *slowly* works your muscle and is an important part of the exercise, not just lifting your forearm up.

What's the best way to time my eating around my workouts?

The timing of food and your exercise routine is an important one. How much food you consume in a sitting determines how long you should wait before you exercise. If you eat a large meal and workout too soon afterwards, you'll feel sluggish and may experience indigestion and nausea. A good rule of thumb is to wait about 3-4 hours after a big meal before engaging in exercise and waiting about 2-3 hours after a medium sized meal. If you have a very small meal or snack it's fine to workout 30 minutes to an hour afterwards. In the **28 Day Plan**, your meals aren't large enough to warrant waiting 3-4 hours. This allows you a bigger window of opportunity to exercise during the day without worrying about timing your meals. As far as timing your post-work snack, I recommend eating something that contains a lot of protein and some carbohydrates to help rebuild tissues and aid in your body's recovery right after you workout. Eating within that first hour of exercising also helps to replace your body's glycogen stores. Keep something healthy in your gym bag or car so you have it available for your post-workout snack.

Will I have to continue working out for the rest of my life to maintain the body I want?

Will you have to wash your hair for the rest of your life? Or brush your teeth? Nothing comes easy, especially when it comes to aging and trying to maintain a healthy weight and staying in shape. Exercise needs to be a part of your life forever to maintain a good weight and to stay healthy. Exercise should be something that you enjoy doing and not just something you *have* to do. It will help you in the long run as well as immediately. You'll age more gracefully, be able to lead a more active life, and prevent health ailments down the road. Once you've gotten into the habit of exercising you'll become addicted and the thought of giving it up won't cross your mind. You can however, reduce your strength training to two days a week instead of three days once you have established the muscle tone you want. It takes at least three days to build the muscles you desire and at least two days to maintain.

I'm having a hard time staying motivated to workout. Any suggestions?

• *Finding a workout partner will help you stay committed to your routine. Knowing that some-one is counting on you to show up to exercise will keep you on track. It can be a friend or even your spouse. Recruit someone to workout with and help each other attain your goals.*

• *If you plan to exercise in the morning, lay out your workout clothes and shoes the night before. This little trick helps you get one step closer to working out. It's a visual reminder of what you know you should do and prevents you from using the excuse that you couldn't find your workout clothes or shoes during the crazy morning rush. It's also helpful in keeping your spouse asleep since you won't be rummaging around trying to get your clothes together if you workout before the family wakes up.*

• *If you workout during your lunch break or right after work, pack your gym clothes and have it ready to go by the door the night before.*

• *If you're a stay-at-home mom with little children, put on your walking or running clothes first thing in the morning. A lot of times moms with small children never know how the day is going to shake out, but if you're ready to go for a walk or a run at a moment's notice, it'll allow you to take advantage of a break in your day whenever it may come. This could be pushing your child in a jogger during his nap time or right when your husband walks in the door after work.*

• *Keep a picture of someone who you find motivating or a picture of yourself when you were at your ideal weight and put it on your fridge, bathroom mirror, or on your desk to help remind you of what you're working towards.*

• *If on a certain day you feel too tired to complete a full workout, tell yourself you're only going to walk or run for just 10 minutes. This makes it seem less challenging and once you get going your adrenalin will kick in and odds are you'll complete a full workout.*

• *If you have the funds to hire a personal trainer, do it. Having someone help you through a workout can be very beneficial because she can customize your workout specifically for your body type, hold you accountable, and give you some extra motivation.*

• *Visualize how you'll look at your weight goal as you're working out to help keep you going. Telling yourself that you **can** achieve your goals while completing your workout will help you get through it. A positive attitude goes a long way!*

• *Keep a calendar designated for recording the days you workout in a visible place. Circle the days that you workout with a marker and record what you did and for how long. For example, I'll write down "weights, 30/40" on days that I lifted weights and ran for 30 minutes with a 5 minute warm up and a 5 minute cool down totaling 40 minutes of cardio. This allows me to see exactly what I've done on which days. It's also a motivator to see how much you can increase your cardio over time. Find a simple system that works for you. Seeing how many days you've exercised is a great motivator. It's also a great visual reminder of what you've done compared to what your goals are. I hang my workout calendar in my bathroom so every morning and night I can see if I'm exercising the amount of days I've challenged myself to. It's also reward-ing to see a lot of days marked showing I'm being disciplined and doing what I know I should to stay healthy and in good shape.*

I travel a lot and find it hard to fit exercise in my schedule when I'm away from home. What do you suggest?

No matter where you are, there's always a way to sneak in some exercise. Most hotels have gyms on site and going for a run or a walk is a great way to get to experience a new city. Take your workout clothes on your trip and make time to get some form of exercise in. If there's not a gym on site or you don't like to workout around other people, purchase a resistance band that easily fits into your luggage. I take this with me whenever I go on vacation because it's small, light weight, and allows me to complete a great workout in the comfort of my hotel room if a gym isn't available. Also, there are many exercises that don't require any equipment and can be done anywhere.

I don't feel like I'm getting the results I should. Could I be doing something wrong?

First, really analyze your food journal to see if you're restricting your caloric intake to what it should be. If you are, maybe you need to reduce the calories you're consuming as long as you don't go below 1200 calories a day. It would be very surprising if you're only eating 1200 calo-ries a day, working out and NOT see any results. Sometimes it takes a person up to two weeks before seeing results, but after that time it would be highly unlikely to not lose any weight. If you're eating only 1200 calories with three meals and two snacks and aren't losing weight, look at your workout routine. Are you really following the **28 Day Plan** like you should? If so, then add to the amount of time or the intensity of your cardio workout and consider if you're ready to increase the weights you're working with. If you can easily complete a set while strength training, it's time to increase the amount you're using. If you're weights are at the poundage you want to keep them, increase the amount of reps you perform. I recommend increasing the weight load first if you haven't received the results you're after. Increasing the amount of reps you complete without increasing poundage is recommended only when you've attained the muscle tone you want.

For some people it takes longer to see results. If you've analyzed everything I've mentioned and know you're following the **28 Day Plan** properly, then it's just a matter of time before you see the results. You know that slacking off on the program won't help you lose the weight, so persevere and it'll happen. Sometimes people feel like they're not seeing any results and then all of a sudden it's as if the pounds just melt off. Every person's body is different so stay on track and you'll reap the rewards of your hard work.

How often should I weigh myself?

Some people have different opinions on this. I read in one publication where it suggested that women only weigh once a month, seven days after their menstrual cycle, to get an accurate reading of their weight. I don't feel that gives you much reaction time. I understand that a woman's weight fluctuates around her cycles but you'll start to see a pattern if you weigh regularly. If you see your weight go up a couple of pounds right before you start your menstrual cycle, you know that's just a part of what happens to your body that time of the month. Seven days after you cycle *does* give you an accurate reading of your weight, but the rest of the month should stay pretty consistent until that week before and during your cycle.

I recommend weighing twice a week on the same two days as you're trying to lose weight. Tuesdays and Friday are usually good days to check your weight. Once you've reached your weight goal, weighing once week can ensure that you're staying on track to help you maintain your goal. Pick one day during the week to weigh; I prefer to weigh on Wednesdays. This way your body has a chance to recover from any of the weekend festivities you might have taken part in, and will give you a pretty accurate reading. Mondays are an awful day to weigh because most of us aren't as strict on the foods and beverages we consume during the weekend. Why make it harder on yourself by choosing that day to weigh in? Seeing the numbers on the scale go down can be very motivating. If your weight doesn't go down as fast as you want, don't get frustrated. It'll happen. You know your mind set and if you'll get frustrated by not seeing results every time you step on the scale, weigh only once a week. If you get excited and motivated by a fraction of a pound lost, then weigh two or three times a week.

Now that I've lost the weight I want, what do I do to keep it off?

This is an exciting place to be! The feeling of knowing your weight and body is right where you want it to be is freeing and makes you feel great. Now, the key is to keep you at that weight. Follow these steps to maintain your goal weight:

1. *Recalculate your daily caloric needs using your new weight so you know how many calories you can consume to maintain the weight you want. (This formula can be found in **Chapter 3 - Knowing Your Numbers.**)*

2. *Continue to record how many calories and fat grams you consume until you adjust to your new caloric needs. It's a mistake to abandon this weight-loss secret as soon as you hit your* goal. Continue to count and record calories until you're very comfortable in knowing how many calories you can consume a day to maintain your weight goal.

3. If you see your weight on the scale go up, start back on the **28 Day Plan** until your weight gets back to where you want it. Of course you'll fluctuate a few pounds up or down throughout the month as mentioned earlier, but when you see the scale stay up, you know it's time to tighten up on your eating habits again.

4. If you're happy with the tone of your body you can reduce your strength training to just two days a week to maintain your muscle tone. If you're like me, you'll want to stick to three days a week because with the hectic life of being a mother, your schedule can be unpredictable. I like to plan for three days of strength training every week because I know situations such as kids being sick, their activities at school and in sports, and work can prevent me from working out. This way I feel like I'm stacking the odds in my favor.

5. Don't let up on your cardio workout. In fact, you might even want to increase it. The more physically fit you become, the less effect a moderate workout can have on your body. Either increase the time you exercise, or increase the intensity. This is even more important if you opt to reduce your strength training to just two days a week.

6. Remember to understand that you're changing your eating and exercise routine permanently. It's more of a lifestyle change and not a "diet" that is to be abandoned once you hit your weight goal. You can have your occasional indulgencies but must always return to your new eating habits to keep off the weight for good. If you've worked hard to reach your goals you certainly don't want go backwards. Stick with your new habits and look and feel your best for life!

CHAPTER 9

EASY, DIET-FRIENDLY RECIPES FOR YOU AND YOUR FAMILY:

APPETIZERS

Stuffed Mushrooms

Preparation Time: 20 minutes   Cooking Time: 10 minutes
Serves: 6

- 1 (10 oz) pkg frozen chopped spinach
- 1 1/2 pounds large fresh mushrooms (about 20)
- 1/4 cup onion, chopped
- 2 cloves garlic, minced
- 1 Tbsp Smart Balance Butter Spread
- 1 1/4 cup Parmesan cheese, grated
- 1/4 cup fine dry bread crumbs
- 4 oz pimiento, finely chopped
- 1/2 tsp dried basil, crushed
- 1/2 tsp dried oregano, crushed
- 1/4 tsp salt
- Pepper to taste

--> Thaw spinach; drain well by squeezing excess liquid out with a paper towel. Spray a baking pan with non-stick spray; set aside.
--> Remove stems from mushrooms and set tops aside. Chop mushroom stems to make 2 cups.
--> Cook chopped mushroom stems, onion, and garlic in butter till onion is just tender. Add thawed spinach and cook over low heat till most of liquid is evaporated.
--> Stir Parmesan cheese, bread crumbs, pimiento, basil, oregano, salt, and pepper into spinach mixture. Spoon mixture into mushroom tops.
--> Place stuffed mushrooms on baking pan. Bake at 425°F for about 10-15 minutes or till mushrooms are tender.

Stuffed Mushrooms

Grocery List:
1 (10 oz) package frozen chopped spinach
1 1⁄2 pounds large fresh mushrooms (about 20)
Onion
2 cloves garlic
Smart Balance Butter Spread
1⁄4 cup grated Parmesan cheese
Dry bread crumbs
4 oz pimiento, finely chopped
Dried basil, crushed
Dried oregano, crushed

Tip: Mushrooms are 80 – 90% water and very low in calories. They have many health benefits including giving your immune system a boost to prevent illness.

Per mushroom: Calories 30, Total Fat 1g, Sodium 93mg, Carbohydrate 4g, Protein 2g, Fiber 3.2g

Oven-Fried Vegetables

Preparation Time: 10 minutes   Cook Time: 9 minutes
Serves: 4

- 1/4 cup fine dry bread crumbs
- 1 Tbsp Parmesan cheese, grated
- 1/8 tsp paprika
- 2 cups 1/4 inch-thick zucchini slices, onion rings, and
    cauliflower florets
- 2 Tbsp low-fat Italian salad dressing

--> Spray a baking sheet with non-stick cooking spray; set aside.

--> In a 9-inch pie plate stir together bread crumbs, Parmesan
    cheese, and paprika. In a medium mixing bowl place zucchini,
    onion rings, and cauliflower. Drizzle vegetables with salad
    dressing and toss till coated. Roll vegetables in crumb mixture.

--> Place vegetables in a single layer on baking sheet. Bake
    vegetables at 450°F for 9-11 minutes or till golden.

Grocery List:
Fine dry bread crumbs
Grated Parmesan cheese
Paprika
2 cups zucchini slices, onion rings, and cauliflower florets
Low-fat Italian salad dressing

 Tip: Buying a good Parmesan cheese and grating it yourself will make your recipes taste better than using pre-grated cheese. The extra time will be worth it when you want your dish to taste its best.

Per serving: Calories 51, Total Fat 2.5g, Sodium 79 mg, Carbohydrate 7g, Protein 2g, Fiber 3.1g

Smokey Salmon Spread

<u>Preparation Time:</u> 5 minutes   <u>Cook Time:</u> 0

<u>Serves:</u> 6-8   <u>Chill Time:</u> 6 hours

- 6 oz low-fat cream cheese, softened
- 2 Tbsp lemon juice
- 1 tsp horseradish
- 2 tsp grated onion
- 1/2 tsp liquid smoke seasoning
- 1 (14.75 oz) sockeye salmon, canned
- 1/4 cup finely chopped fresh parsley

--> Combine all but salmon.

--> Drain salmon and stir into cream cheese mixture. Refrigerate 6 hours or overnight.

--> Serve with low-fat bagel chips or cracker of choice.

Grocery List:

6 oz low-fat cream cheese
Lemon juice
Horseradish
Onion
Liquid smoke seasoning
1 (14.75 oz) sockeye salmon, canned
Fresh parsley

Tip: *Eating the bones in canned salmon might sound gross, but it actually gives you a large dose of calcium. When the bones and salmon are mixed together, you won't even realize you're eating them and will be getting their added health benefit.*

Per serving: Calories 159, Total Fat 11g, Sodium 341mg, Carbohydrate 0g, Protein 12g, Fiber 0g

Pickled Shrimp

Preparation Time: 10 minutes
Cook Time: **3** minutes
Serves: **8**
Chill Time: **24** hours

- 1 pound fresh shrimp
- 2 large Bermuda onions, cut in rings
- 2 large green peppers, cut in rings
- 1 (16 oz) bottle low-fat Catalina French Dressing
- 1 (10 oz) bottle vinegar
- Pepper to taste

--> Place shrimp in a pot of boiling water and boil for 3 minutes. Drain in a colander and rinse with cold water. Peel and set aside.

--> Alternately layer shrimp, onion rings, and pepper rings in a container with a tight seal.

--> Pour dressing and vinegar over shrimp and vegetables. Sprinkle with black pepper.

--> Seal container and marinate for 24 hours. Shake container or stir occasionally to mix.

--> Drain off liquid and serve in a large bowl with toothpicks.

Grocery List:
1 pound fresh shrimp
2 large Bermuda onions
2 large green peppers
1 (16 oz) bottle low-fat Catalina French Dressing
1 (10 oz) bottle vinegar

 Tip: You can also add mushrooms, cauliflower or artichoke hearts.

Per serving: Calories 157, Total Fat 7g, Sodium 266mg, Carbohydrate 16g, Protein 12g, Fiber 1.5g

Creamy Hummus

<u>Preparation Time:</u> 5 minutes   <u>Cook Time:</u> 0 minutes

<u>Serves:</u> 16

- 1 (15 oz) can chick peas, drained reserving liquid
- 1/4 cup olive oil
- 3 garlic cloves
- 1 1/2 Tbsp lemon juice
- 3/4 tsp cumin, ground
- 1/2 cup fresh Italian parsley, stemmed and chopped
- Salt and pepper to taste

--> Place garlic and parsley in a food processor and chop fine.

--> Add chick peas, olive oil, salt, pepper, cumin, and lemon juice. Process until smooth. Use bean liquid to thin if desired.

--> Serve with vegetables, baked tortillas, or toasted pita chips.

Grocery List:

15 oz can chick peas
Olive oil
3 garlic cloves
Lemon juice
Ground cumin
Fresh Italian parsley

Per serving: Calories 64, Total Fat 4g,
Sodium 104mg, Carbohydrate 7g,
Protein 2g, Fiber 1g

BREAKFAST

Asparagus Frittata

Preparation Time: 15 minutes   Cooking Time: 10 minutes
Serves: 4

- 3/4 pound fresh asparagus spears
- 6 eggs
- 3/4 cup low-fat cottage cheese
- 2 tsp prepared mustard
- 1/8 tsp salt
- Dash black pepper
- 1 cup fresh mushrooms, sliced
- 1 small tomato, cut into wedges

--> Cook fresh asparagus spears in microwave with 1 Tbsp water for 2-3 minutes until crisp-tender; set aside.

--> Meanwhile, in a medium mixing bowl beat eggs till foamy. Beat in cottage cheese, mustard, salt, and pepper; set aside.

--> Spray a 10-inch ovenproof skillet with non-stick cooking spray. Cook mushrooms over medium heat till just tender. Stir in asparagus reserving 3 spears for garnish. Pour egg mixture over mushrooms and asparagus. Place the 3 spears on the center.

--> Cook mixture over low heat about 5 minutes or till mixture bubbles slightly and begins to set around the edges.

--> Bake frittata, uncovered at 400°F for about 10 minutes or till set. Complete garnish by placing tomato wedges and asparagus on top.

Grocery List:
3/4 pound fresh asparagus spears
6 eggs
3/4 cup low-fat cottage cheese
Prepared mustard
1 cup fresh mushrooms, sliced
1 small tomato

Per serving: Calories 183, Total Fat 10g, Sodium 375mg, Carbohydrate 7g, Protein 18g, Fiber 1.1g

Breakfast Turkey Patties

<u>Preparation Time:</u> 5 minutes   <u>Cook Time:</u> 10 minutes

<u>Serves:</u> 4

- 1 pound lean ground turkey
- 1/2 tsp salt
- 1/2 tsp dried sage leaves
- 1/2 tsp black pepper
- 1/4 tsp ground ginger
- 1/4 tsp cayenne pepper

--> Crumble turkey in a large bowl. Add salt, sage, pepper, ginger, and cayenne. Shape into 8 patties.

--> In a large skillet, cook patties over medium-heat for 5 minutes on each side or until meat is not longer pink.

Grocery List:
1 pound lean ground turkey
Dried sage leaves
Ground ginger
Cayenne pepper

Tip: This dish is so good I like to serve it for dinner with brown rice and vegetables.

Per serving: Calories 85, Total Fat 5g, Sodium 295mg, Carbohydrate .5g, Protein 10g, Fiber .5g

Spinach and Mushroom Omelet

Preparation Time: 10 minutes   **Cook Time:** 8-10 minutes

Serves: 4

- 2 eggs
- 6 egg whites
- 2 Tbsp Parmesan cheese, grated
- 2 Tbsp cheddar cheese, shredded
- 1/4 tsp salt
- 1/4 tsp crushed red pepper flakes
- 1/4 tsp garlic powder
- 1/4 tsp freshly ground black pepper
- 1 cup fresh mushrooms, sliced
- 4 Tbsp green pepper, finely chopped
- 2 Tbsp onion, finely chopped
- 1 tsp olive oil
- 2 cups torn fresh spinach

--> In a small bowl, beat eggs and egg whites. Add cheeses, salt, pepper flakes, garlic powder and pepper; mix well and set aside.

--> In an 8" non-stick skillet, sauté mushrooms, green peppers, and onion in oil for 4-5 minutes or until tender. Add spinach; cook and stir until wilted.

--> Add egg mixture. As eggs set, lift edges, letting uncooked portion flow underneath. Cut into wedges and serve immediately.

Grocery List:

8 eggs
Grated Parmesan cheese
Cheddar cheese, shredded
Crushed red pepper flakes
Garlic powder
1 cup fresh mushrooms, sliced
Green pepper
Onion
Olive oil
2 cups fresh spinach

Per serving: Calories 110, Total Fat 6g, Sodium 489mg, Carbohydrate 4g, Protein 11g, Fiber 1g

Peach Smoothies

Preparation Time: 5 minutes   _Cook Time:_ 0 minutes

Serves: 4

- 1 cup peach or apricot nectar
- 1 cup fresh or frozen peaches, sliced
- 1/2 cup fat-free vanilla yogurt
- 4 ice cubes

--> In a blender, combine all ingredients. Cover and process until blended.

--> Pour into chilled glasses and serve.

Grocery List:

1 cup peach or apricot nectar
1 cup fresh or frozen peaches, sliced
1/2 cup fat-free vanilla yogurt

Tip: Sometimes good fresh peaches are hard to find. They're a very perishable food and many times are heavily gassed to help prolong their shelf life. If the peaches don't have a sweet smell and aren't slightly soft, you might be better off buying them frozen to ensure the best flavor.

Per serving: Calories 120, Total Fat .5g,
Sodium 29mg, Carbohydrate 29g,
Protein 2g, Fiber 2g

The Perfect Smoothie

Preparation Time: 5 minutes   Cook Time: 0 minutes

Serves: 5

- 2 ripe bananas
- 1 cup low-fat plain yogurt
- 1 cup fresh or frozen blueberries
- 1 cup fresh or frozen strawberries (without syrup)
- 1 cup skim milk
- 2 Tbsp wheat germ (optional)

(If you use fresh berries instead of frozen you might want to add 1-2 cups of ice to chill.)

--> Mix in a blender until smooth. To thin mixture add ice or milk.

Grocery List:

2 ripe bananas
1 cup low-fat plain yogurt
1 cup fresh or frozen blueberries
1 cup fresh or frozen strawberries *(without syrup if frozen)*
1 cup skim milk
Wheat germ *(optional)*

Tip: This recipe is a great way to make use of bananas that are too ripe to eat. You can even peel overripe bananas and place in an air-tight bag or container in the freezer to use whenever you're in the mood for a smoothie.

Per serving: Calories 125, Total Fat 1g, Sodium 67mg, Carbohydrate 23g, Protein 5g, Fiber 2.5g

SOUPS & SALADS

MC's Heart-Healthy Salad

Preparation Time: 10 minutes   **Cook Time:** 0 minutes

Serves: 6

- 2 cups mixed greens
- 2 cups Romaine Lettuce
- 1 tomato, chopped
- 6 radishes, chopped
- 1/2 red onion, chopped
- 1 large carrot or 6 baby carrots, chopped
- 1 cucumber, sliced
- 1/4 head red cabbage, thinly sliced
- 1/2 red bell pepper, chopped
- 1/4 cup pine nuts
- Your choice of fat-free salad dressing

--> Toss vegetables together and serve with dressing on the side.

Grocery List:

Mixed greens
Romaine lettuce
1 tomato
Radishes
1 large carrot or 6 small baby carrots
Cucumber
Red cabbage
Red bell pepper
Pine nuts
Your choice of fat-free salad dressing

Per serving: Calories 60, Total Fat 2.5g,
Sodium 16mg, Carbohydrate 7g, Protein 2.6g,
Fiber 2.3g *(not including dressing)*

MC's Heart-Healthy Salad with Chicken Strips

Preparation Time: 12 minutes   Cook Time: 10-15 minutes
Serves: 6

- 1 pound boneless, skinless chicken breast, cut into strips
- All-purpose seasoning to taste
- Pepper to taste
- 2 cups mixed greens
- 2 cups Romaine Lettuce
- 1 tomato, chopped
- 6 radishes, chopped
- 1/2 red onion, chopped
- 1 large carrot or 6 baby carrots, chopped
- 1 cucumber, sliced
- 1/4 head red cabbage, thinly sliced
- 1/2 red bell pepper, chopped
- 1/4 cup pine nuts
- Your choice of fat-free salad dressing

--> Spray a skillet with non-stick cooking spray and heat.
    Add chicken strips, seasoning, pepper and cook over medium-
    high heat, turning once, until chicken is no longer pink.
--> While chicken is cooking, mix remaining ingredients.
--> Let chicken cool and place on salad.
--> Serve with dressing on the side.

Grocery List:

1 pound boneless, skinless chicken breasts
All-purpose seasoning
Mixed greens
Romaine lettuce
1 tomato
Radishes
1 large carrot or 6 small baby carrots
Cucumber
Red cabbage
Red bell pepper
Pine nuts

Choice of fat-free salad dressing

Per serving: Calories 143, Total Fat 3.5g,
Sodium 66mg, Carbohydrate 7g,
Protein 20g, Fiber 2.3g (not including dressing)

Power Vegetable Soup

_Preparation Time_: 15 - 20 minutes   _Cook Time_: 30 minutes
Makes: 20 cups

- 20 oz extra lean ground turkey
- 3 Tbsp Worcestershire sauce
- 1 large sweet onion, chopped
- 1 pkg (16 oz) frozen butter beans
- 1 pkg (16 oz) frozen corn
- 2 (14 1/2 oz) can tomatoes and okra
- 2 large carrots, sliced
- 1/2 head cabbage, chopped
- 46 oz reduced-sodium V8 Juice
- 3 cups of water
- 1/2 tsp black pepper
- 1/4 - 1/2 tsp cayenne pepper

--> Brown ground turkey with onions and Worcestershire sauce

--> Mix all ingredients, except seasoning, in a large stock pot and bring to a boil.

--> Cover on simmer for 30 minutes, stirring occasionally.

--> Add black and cayenne pepper and cook for 15 more minutes.

(This recipe freezes well. Make the most of your time by freezing some for later.)

Grocery List:

20 oz extra lean ground turkey
Worcestershire sauce
1 large sweet onion
1 pkg (16 oz) frozen butter beans
1 pkg (16 oz) frozen corn
2 (14 1/2 oz) can tomatoes and okra
2 large carrots
1/2 head cabbage
46 oz reduced-sodium _V8 Juice_
Black pepper
Cayenne pepper

Per serving: Calories 143, Total Fat 1g, Sodium 281mg, Carbohydrate 20g, Protein 11g, Fiber 11g

Lentil Soup with Vegetables

<u>Preparation Time</u>: 15 minutes   <u>Cook Time</u>: 1 hour

<u>Makes</u>: 9 cups

- 2 cups brown lentils
- 1 Tbsp olive oil
- 1 large onion, chopped
- 2 stalks celery, chopped
- 2 cloves garlic, finely chopped
- 8 oz parsnip or turnip, chopped
- 2 large carrots, chopped
- 2 Qt vegetable stock (reduced-sodium, or 1 QT stock mixed
  with 1 QT water)
- 1 Tbsp tomato paste
- 1/4 tsp dried thyme
- 1 bay leaf
- 1/8 tsp pepper

--> Rinse lentils in a colander. In a large saucepan, heat oil over medium heat.

--> Add onion, celery, and garlic and sauté, stirring constantly, about 5-7 minutes until softened and golden brown.

--> Add turnips or parsnip, carrots, then 1/4 cup of stock and cook, stirring frequently, until slightly soft.

--> Bring to a boil then simmer, partially covered & stir occasionally, about 50 minutes, until lentils and vegetables are soft.

--> Add pepper. Remove bay leaf and discard before serving.

Lentil Soup with Vegetables

Grocery List:
2 cups brown lentils
Olive oil
1 large onion
2 stalks celery
2 cloves garlic
8 ounces parsnip or turnip
2 large carrots
2 quarts vegetable stock *(reduced-sodium, or 1 QT stock mixed with 1 QT water)*
Tomato paste (small can)
Dried thyme
1 bay leaf

Tip: Lentils might be small in size, but they're big in nutrients. Lentils are packed with dietary fiber, folate, magnesium, iron and protein.

Per serving: Calories 217, Total Fat 3g, Sodium 178mg, Carbohydrate 35g, Protein 15g, Fiber 8g

White Bean Soup with Carrots

Preparation Time: 10 minutes plus soak time
Cook Time: 1 3/4 hours   Makes: 8 cups

- 2 cups dried navy beans, washed and picked over
- 1 Tbsp olive oil
- 1 large onion, sliced
- 6 garlic cloves, coarsely chopped
- 6 cups vegetable stock (reduced-sodium or 3 cups stock with 3 cups water)
- 2 large carrots, sliced
- 1 Tbsp chopped fresh sage or 1/2 tsp dried sage, crumbled
- 1/8 tsp pepper
- Snipped basil to garnish if desired

--> Place beans in a large saucepan and generously cover with water. Bring to a boil and let boil for 2 minutes, then remove from heat. Allow to soak at least 1 hour or overnight.

--> Drain beans, rinse thoroughly under cold water, and drain again.

--> In a large saucepan, heat oil over medium heat. Add onion, garlic, and 2 Tbsp stock, and sauté about 5 minutes, until softened but not brown.

--> Add carrots and sage, stirring for about 2 minutes.

--> Add soaked beans and remaining stock and bring to a boil. Simmer soup, partially covered and stir occasionally, about 1 1/2 hours, until the beans are quite tender.

--> Remove soup from heat. Transfer 1 1/2 cups of the beans and vegetables to a blender or food processor and puree until smooth. Add 1/2 cup of liquid and process to combine.

--> Return puree to soup and add pepper. Heat and simmer soup 3 minutes longer.

White Bean Soup with Carrots

Grocery List:

2 cups dried navy beans
Olive oil
1 large onion
6 garlic cloves
6 cups vegetable stock *(reduced sodium or 3 cups stock with 3 cups water)*
2 large carrots
Fresh sage or 1/2 tsp dried sage, crumbled
Fresh basil to garnish, if desired

Tip: Did you know that baby carrots are really just the center of regular carrots? A farmer in California got tired of throwing out all of the imperfect carrots and decided to try to make good use of the waste. He revolutionized the carrot industry by cutting each carrot into 2 segments and then shaving the skin off around the carrot creating the baby carrot as we know it today.

Per serving: Calories 136, Total Fat 2g, Sodium 196mg, Carbohydrate 24g, Protein 6g, Fiber 5g

Julianne's Cole Slaw

<u>Preparation Time:</u> 5 minutes   <u>Cook Time:</u> 0 minutes
<u>Marinate time:</u> 4-6 hours   <u>Serves:</u> 10

- 1-2 Tbsp white vinegar (may also use hot pepper vinegar)
- 1/2 tsp salt
- 1/4 tsp black pepper
- 1 medium head cabbage
- 1/2 cup yellow onion, finely chopped
- 3 Tbsp Low-fat Hellman's Mayonnaise

--> Remove outer leaves of cabbage; wash and pat dry. Quarter cabbage; slice cabbage on an angle. (How you slice the cabbage is important.)

--> Add vinegar, onion, salt and pepper. Toss; cover and refrigerate until chilled or about 2 hours.

--> Add mayonnaise and toss until all cabbage is coated. Let chill 4-6 hours.

Grocery List:

White or hot pepper vinegar
1 yellow onion
Head of cabbage
Low-fat Hellman's mayonnaise

Tip: Cabbage develops a bitter taste around its core, so make sure not to cut too close to it to protect the flavor of your cole slaw.

Per serving: Calories 40, Total Fat 1.5g, Sodium 168mg, Carbohydrate 5.3g, Protein 0g, Fiber 2.1g

Lentil, Garbanzo Bean and Tomato Salad

Preparation Time: 10 minutes   Cook Time: 25 minutes

Serves: 4   Chill Time: 4 hours

- 1 cup lentils
- 2 large carrots, peeled and diced
- 1 bay leaf
- 2 1/2 cups water
- 1 can garbanzo beans (chick peas), rinsed and drained
- 1/2 basket grape tomatoes, halved
- 1 cup fresh parsley, chopped
- 5 green onions, chopped
- 1/2 cup red onion, chopped
- 3 Tbsp olive oil
- 2 1/2 Tbsp fresh lemon juice
- Salt and pepper to taste

--> Combine water, lentils, diced carrots, and bay leaf in a medium saucepan and bring to a boil. Reduce heat, cover and simmer until lentils are just tender, about 25 minutes.

--> Drain; transfer to a large bowl and cool.

--> Mix all remaining ingredients into lentil mixture. Gently stir until well blended; cover and refrigerate. Stir before serving.

Grocery List:

1 cup lentils
2 large carrots
1 bay leaf
1 can garbanzo beans (chick peas)
1/2 basket grape tomatoes
1 cup fresh parsley
5 green onions

1/2 cup red onion
Olive oil
Lemon

Per serving: Calories 250, Total Fat 8.5g,
Sodium 50mg, Carbohydrate 34g,
Protein 13.5g, Fiber 14g

Greek Salad

Preparation Time: 10 minutes   Cook Time: 0 minutes
Serves: 4

- 4 cups torn red leaf lettuce
- 1 large tomato, cut into wedges
- 8 cucumber slices, halved
- 4 radishes, sliced
- 2 red onion slices, quartered
- 4 Tbsp ripe olives, sliced
- 2 Tbsp feta cheese, crumbled

Dressing:
- 2 Tbsp red wine vinegar
- 4 tsp water
- 4 tsp olive oil
- 2 garlic cloves, minced
- 1/2 tsp sugar
- 1/4 tsp salt
- 1/8 tsp black pepper

--> In a small bowl, combine lettuce, tomato, cucumber, radishes, onion, olives, and feta cheese.

--> In a jar with a tight fitting lid, combine the dressing ingredients; shake well. Drizzle over salad and toss to coat. Serve immediately.

Grocery List:
Red leaf lettuce
1 large tomato
1 cucumber
4 radishes
1 red onion
4 Tbsp ripe olives
2 Tbsp feta cheese, crumbled

Dressing:
Red wine vinegar
Olive oil
2 garlic cloves, minced
Sugar

Per serving: Calories 89, Total Fat 6g, Sodium 265mg, Carbohydrate 7g, Protein 2g, Fiber 2g

Fruit Salad

<u>Preparation Time:</u> 10 minutes   <u>Cook Time:</u> 0 minutes
<u>Serves:</u> 10 – 1/2 cup servings   <u>Chill Time:</u> 4 hours

- 2 cups fresh strawberries, sliced
- 2 cups red grapes, halved
- 1 small cantaloupe, cut into chunks
- 2 medium firm bananas, sliced
- 1/3 cup of orange juice

--> In a large bowl, combine all fruit. Pour juice over fruit and toss to coat.
--> Cover and refrigerate for 4 hours. Stir just before serving.

Grocery List:
2 cups fresh strawberries
2 cups red grapes
1 small cantaloupe
2 medium firm bananas
Orange juice

Tip: Choose a cantaloupe that's yellow and has a sweet smell. Odds are that if the cantaloupe doesn't smell sweet, it won't taste sweet. Never refrigerate cantaloupe unless you've already cut it.

Per serving: Calories 63, Total Fat .5g, Sodium 5mg, Carbohydrate 15g, Protein 1g, Fiber 2g

Tuna Salad

Preparation Time: 5 minutes   Cook Time: 0 minutes
Serves: 3

- 1 can tuna in water, drained
- 1 Tbsp low-fat mayonnaise
- 1 celery stalk, chopped
- 1 medium carrot, chopped
- 2 Tbsp sweet relish, drained
- 1 tsp prepared mustard
- Black pepper and garlic power to taste

--> Mix all ingredients and serve.

Grocery List:
1 can tuna in water
Low-fat mayonnaise
1 stalk celery
1 medium carrot
Sweet relish

Tip: *Be careful how much tuna you eat per week. Tuna is high in mercury and if consumed in large quantities, it can have adverse effects on your health. Albacore has about 3 times the amount of mercury than chunk tuna. Even though the exact amount of tuna you can consume is not known, most agree that limiting yourself to 1/2 - 1 can of Albacore tuna and 1 – 2 cans of chunk tuna per week will keep the mercury at a safe level with no risks. Tuna has its benefits so don't shy away from it; just limit how much you consume.*

Per serving: Calories 87, Total Fat 2g, Sodium 325mg, Carbohydrate 5g, Protein 11g, Fiber 0g

ENTREES

Baked Parmesan Salmon

Preparation Time: 10 minutes   _Cook Time:_ 20-30 minutes
Serves: 4

- 4 (4 oz) salmon fillets
- 1/3 Low-fat mayonnaise
- 3 Tbsp grated Parmesan cheese (freshly grated is best)
- 2 Tbsp green onions OR fresh chives, sliced
- 1/2 tsp white wine
- Dash of Worcestershire sauce

--> Rinse salmon and pat dry. Spray a baking dish with nonstick cooking spray and place fillets skin side down.

--> In a small bowl, stir together mayonnaise, Parmesan cheese, green onions, wine and Worcestershire sauce. Spread mixture over fish.

--> Bake, uncovered, at 350° for 20-30 minutes or until fish flakes easily with a fork. Do not overcook.

Grocery List:
4 (4 oz) salmon fillets
Low-fat mayonnaise
Parmesan cheese
Green onions or fresh chives
White wine
Worcestershire sauce

Per serving: Calories 135, Total Fat 10g,
Sodium 262mg, Carbohydrate 1.4g,
Protein 7.7g, Fiber 0g

Turkey Burgers

<u>Preparation Time:</u> 5 minutes   <u>Cook Time:</u> 15 minutes
<u>Serves:</u> 4

- 1 pound extra-lean, or lean ground turkey*
- 2 Tbsp Worcestershire sauce
- 1 tsp garlic powder
- Salt and pepper to taste

--> Mix all ingredients and shape into patties.
--> Grill over medium-high heat for about 7-8 minutes on each
    side or in a skillet sprayed with nonstick cooking spray for
    about 15-20 minutes until cooked through.

* extra-lean ground turkey is difficult to grill so if you use it,
  add a little applesauce to the patties to make them moist.

(This recipe tastes great with the Simple Mushrooms
and Onions served on top of the burger.)

Grocery List:
1 pound lean or extra-lean ground turkey
Worcestershire sauce
Garlic powder

Tip: If you use lean turkey meat instead of extra-lean, wrap
the cooked burger in several paper towels after it's been cooked,
and squeeze out the extra grease to reduce the fat content.
You'll lose the fat but not the flavor.

Per serving *(without a bun):*
Calories 130, Total Fat 1.7g, Sodium 71mg,
Carbohydrate 0g, Protein 27g, Fiber 0g

Slow-Cooked Chicken

Preparation Time: 5 minutes   _Cook Time:_ 4-7 hours in a
Serves: 4   slow-cooker

- 4 medium boneless, skinless chicken breasts
- 1/2 cup water
- All-Purpose Seasoning

--> Place chicken and water in slow cooker and sprinkle with
    seasoning.
--> Cook on low for 4-7 hours or till chicken is no longer pink.

Grocery List:
4 medium boneless, skinless chicken breast
All-purpose seasoning

Tip: To make this recipe easier on your budget, purchase
chicken with the skin on and remove it yourself. It doesn't
take much time to do and can help reduce your grocery bill.

Per serving: Calories130 , Total Fat 1.5g,
Sodium 77mg, Carbohydrate 0g,
Protein 27.2g, Fiber 0g

Honey Mustard Chicken

Preparation Time: 6 minutes   Cooking Time: 7 minutes

Serves: 4

- 4 medium thin boneless, skinless chicken breasts
- 2 tsp prepared mustard
- 2 tsp honey

--> Spray rack of a broiler pan with nonstick cooking spray. Arrange chicken on broiler rack.

--> Broil 4-5 inches from the heat for about 6 minutes.

--> Meanwhile, stir together mustard and honey in a small bowl. Brush over chicken.

--> Broil 1-2 minutes longer or till chicken is tender and no longer pink.

Grocery List:
4 medium boneless skinless chicken breast
Prepared mustard
Honey

Tip: Honey is a great food to add to recipes because it offers sweetness along with many health benefits. Honey has plenty of antioxidents and anti-bacterial properties that fight infections, aid in tissue healing and reduce inflammation and scarring. When you can, substitute honey in places where you use regular sugar to still have a taste of sweetness but with the added health benefits.

Per serving: Calories 153, Total Fat 3g, Sodium 77 mg, Carbohydrate 3g, Protein 26g, Fiber 0g

Sauteed Scallops

Preparation Time: 8 minutes   Cook Time: 3-4 Minutes

Serves: 4

- 1 pound of sea scallops (may also use bay scallops)
- 1 Tbsp olive oil
- 1/2 Tbsp lemon juice
- 2 Tbsp shallots, chopped
- 1 garlic clove, minced
- 2 Tbsp parsley, finely chopped
- 2 Tbsp dry white wine

--> Rinse scallops and pat dry; set aside.

--> Heat oil in a skillet over medium-high heat.

--> Add scallops, shallots, lemon juice and garlic to skillet and cook for 1-2 minutes, stirring frequently.

--> Add wine and continue to cook 2-3 minutes or until scallops are opaque. Sprinkle with parsley and serve.

Grocery List:
1 pound of sea scallops
Olive oil
Lemon juice
Shallots
Fresh parsley
Dry white wine
1 garlic clove

Per serving: Calories 135 , Total Fat 4.5g,
Sodium 160mg, Carbohydrate 3g,
Protein 17g, Fiber 0g

Chicken Marsala

<u>Preparation Time:</u> 11 minutes   <u>Cooking Time:</u> 8 minutes
<u>Serves:</u> 4

- 4 medium boneless, skinless chicken breast halves
- 1 1/2 cups sliced fresh mushrooms
- 2 Tbsp chopped green onion
- 2 Tbsp water
- 1/4 cup dry Marsala or dry sherry
- 1/4 tsp salt
- Nonstick cooking spray

--> Place 1 piece of chicken, thick side up, between 2 pieces of plastic wrap. Working from the center to the edges, pound lightly with a meat mallet to about 1/4 inch thickness. Repeat with remaining chicken pieces.

--> Spray a large skillet with nonstick spray coating. Preheat skillet over medium heat. Add chicken breast halves and cook over medium heat for 3-4 minutes or till tender and no longer pink. Transfer to a platter; keep warm.

--> Add mushrooms, green onions, water, and salt to skillet. Cook over medium heat till mushrooms are tender and most of the liquid has evaporated (about 3 minutes). Add Marsala or dry sherry to skillet and heat through. Spoon vegetables and sauce over chicken and serve.

Grocery List:
4 medium boneless, skinless chicken breast halves
Fresh mushrooms
Green onions
Dry Marsala or dry sherry

Per serving: Calories 216, Total Fat 2g, Sodium 170mg, Carbohydrate 11g, Protein 31g, Fiber 1.6g

Easy Chicken Cacciatore

Preparation Time: 10 minutes   _Cook Time:_ 15 minutes
Serves: 5

- 1 pound of boneless skinless chicken breasts, sliced into strips
- 1 medium green pepper, cut into 1-inch pieces
- 1 small onion, cut into 1-inch pieces
- 1 (15 oz) can seasoned tomato sauce
- 2/3 cup water
- 1/4 tsp pepper
- 1/2 tsp Italian seasoning
- 9 ounces whole wheat angel hair pasta

--> Cook pasta according to package directions, omitting salt and oil.

--> Coat a non-stick skillet with cooking spray and cook over medium heat. Add chicken, green pepper, and onion; sauté until chicken is no longer pink and vegetables are crisp-tender.

--> Stir in tomato sauce, water, pepper and seasonings. Reduce heat and simmer, uncovered, for 5 minutes. Stir often.

--> Serve over cooked wheat pasta.

Grocery List:
1 pound of boneless skinless chicken breasts
1 medium green pepper
1 small onion
1 (15 oz) can seasoned tomato sauce
Italian seasoning
9 oz whole wheat angel hair pasta

Per serving: Calories 416, Total Fat 6g,
Sodium 87mg, Carbohydrate 47g,
Protein 41g, Fiber 5.5g

Szechuan Chicken and Vegetables

Preparation Time: 5 minutes   Cook Time: 8 minutes
Makes: 4 servings

- 2 tsp sesame oil
- 1 pound boneless, skinless chicken breast
- 1/4 tsp dried red pepper flakes
- 10 oz frozen stir-fry vegetables or 2 1/2 cups of fresh broccoli, cauliflower and carrots mixed
- 1/4 cup low-sodium teriyaki sauce

--> Heat oil in a large non-stick skillet over medium heat. Add chicken and sprinkle with pepper flakes; stir-fry 3 minutes.

--> Add vegetables and teriyaki sauce; stir-fry 5 minutes or till vegetables are crisp-tender and chicken is thoroughly cooked.

--> Serve over whole wheat angel hair pasta, or brown rice.

Grocery List:
Sesame oil
1 pound boneless, skinless chicken breast
1/4 tsp dried red pepper flakes
10 oz pkg frozen stir-fry vegetables
   or 2 1/2 cups of fresh broccoli, cauliflower and carrots mixed
Low-sodium teriyaki sauce
Whole wheat angel hair pasta or brown rice

Tip: Szechuan is a style of Chinese cooking that is spicy and usually prepared in oil. You can reduce or increase the amount of red pepper flakes in this recipe to suit your taste.

Per serving: Calories 183, Total Fat 3.7g, Sodium 341mg, Carbohydrate 8g, Protein 29g, Fiber 1.2g (not including pasta or rice)

Citrus-Jerk Orange Roughy

Preparation Time: **3** minutes   Cook Time: **7** minutes

Serves: **4**

- 4 (4 oz) orange roughy fillets
- 4 tsp jerk seasoning
- 1 tsp olive oil
- 4 Tbsp orange marmalade
- 3 Tbsp water
- 2 Tbsp lemon juice
- 1/8 tsp freshly ground black pepper

--> Sprinkle both sides of fillets evenly with seasoning, pressing gently to adhere. Coat a large nonstick skillet with non-stick cooking spray; add oil and place over medium-high heat until hot.

--> Add fillets; cook **3** minutes on each side or until fish flakes easily with a fork. Remove from skillet; set aside, and keep warm.

--> Add orange marmalade and remaining ingredients to skillet. Bring to a boil, and cook 1 minute. Pour sauce over fish, and serve immediately.

Grocery List:
4 (4 oz) orange roughy fillets
Jerk seasoning
Olive oil
Orange marmalade
Lemon juice

Tip: Most kids who don't usually care for fish like Orange Roughy due to it's mild flavor. It's a great fish to use for pickey eaters!

Per serving: Calories 151, Total Fat 2g, Sodium 142mg, Carbohydrate 16g, Protein 17g, Fiber .4g

Barbeque Meatloaf

Preparation Time: 8 minutes   Cook Time: 25-30 minutes
Serves: 4

- 1 pound extra-lean ground turkey, or ground beef
- 1/2 cup barbecue sauce, divided
- 1/4 onion, chopped
- 1/4 cup Italian-seasoned dry breadcrumbs
- 2 egg whites
- 1/4 tsp black pepper

--> Combine meat, 1/4 cup barbecue sauce, onion, breadcrumbs,
    egg whites, and pepper in a large bowl; stir well.
--> Shape mixture into a 7" x 5" loaf on a rack in a roasting pan.
    Spread remaining 1/4 cup barbeque sauce over loaf.
    Bake at 375°F for 30 minutes or until desired doneness.

Grocery List:
1 pound extra-lean ground turkey, or
ground beef
Barbecue sauce
1 yellow onion
Italian-seasoned dry breadcrumbs
Eggs

Tip: *You can make your own breadcrumbs by toasting bread,
letting it get cold and then crumbling it up in a resealable plastic bag.
I like to do this because it's difficult to find whole wheat bread crumbs,
but by using my own whole wheat bread, I can make them myself.*

Per serving: Calories 228, Total Fat 3g
(7g if using 95% lean beef), Sodium 535mg,
Carbohydrate 10g, Protein 28g, Fiber .5g

Pineapple-Chicken and Rice Bake

<u>Preparation Time:</u> 20 minutes   <u>Marinate:</u> 4-24 hours

<u>Serves:</u> 6   <u>Cook Time:</u> 1 hour

- 2 pounds boneless skinless chicken breasts
- 1/2 cup onion, chopped
- 1 large red pepper, cut into squares
- 1 (8 oz) can pineapple chunks
- 1/4 cup frozen orange juice concentrate, thawed
- 2 Tbsp reduced sodium soy sauce
- 1/8 tsp ground cloves
- 2/3 cup brown rice
- 1 cup chicken broth
- Parsley and paprika to garnish

--> Place chicken, onion, and red pepper in a large re-sealable plastic bag.

--> In a small bowl stir together undrained pineapple, orange juice concentrate, soy sauce and cloves. Pour pineapple mixture over chicken in bag then seal. Marinate in the refrigerator for 4-24 hours, turning bag occasionally.

--> Drain chicken, reserving marinade and vegetables. Set chicken aside.

--> Place uncooked rice in a casserole dish approximately 13x9x2". Stir chicken broth and reserved marinade and vegetables into the rice. Top with chicken breasts and cover with foil.

--> Bake at 375°F for about 1 hour or until chicken is no longer pink and rice is tender. Sprinkle with paprika and garnish with parsley.

Grocery List Next Page

Pineapple-Chicken and Rice Bake

Grocery List:

2 pounds boneless, skinless chicken breasts
1 yellow onion
1 large red pepper
1 (8 oz) can pineapple chunks
Frozen orange juice concentrate
Reduced-sodium soy sauce
Ground cloves
Brown rice
Chicken broth
Parsley and paprika to garnish

Tip: *When picking out fresh pineapple choose the one with the sweetest smell and one that's yellow in color. If you aren't going to be using it within a few days, pick out one that is a little green so it doesn't get too ripe.*

Per serving: Calories 280, Total Fat 3g, Sodium 337mg, Carbohydrate 30g, Protein 25g, Fiber 2g

Chicken and Broccoli Casserole

Preparation Time: 20 minutes   Cooking Time: 40 minutes

Serves: 6

- 2 1/2 cups cooked chicken or turkey, chopped
- 4 oz whole wheat medium noodles
- 1 (10 oz) pkg frozen chopped broccoli, thawed
- 1/2 cup sliced green onions
- 1 can of low-fat condensed cream of mushroom soup
- 1/2 cup skim milk
- 1/2 cup Swiss cheese, shredded
- 1 tsp dried basil, crushed
- 1/8 tsp pepper
- Paprika

--> Cook noodles according to package directions. Drain well.

--> In a 2-quart casserole dish stir together noodles, chicken or turkey, broccoli, and green onions.

--> In a medium mixing bowl stir together soup, milk, cheese, basil, and pepper. Stir into noodle mixture.

--> Bake, covered, at 350°F for 40-45 minutes or until thoroughly heated. Sprinkle with paprika and serve.

Grocery List:

2 1/2 cups cooked chicken or turkey, chopped
4 oz whole wheat medium noodles
1 (10 oz) pkg frozen chopped broccoli
Green onions
1 can of low-fat condensed cream of mushroom soup
Skim milk
1/2 cup Swiss cheese, shredded
Dried basil, crushed
Paprika

Per serving: Calories 290, Total Fat 11g,
Sodium 508mg, Carbohydrate 22g,
Protein 25g, Fiber 4.1g

Tex-Mex Turkey Tenderloins

Preparation Time: 10 minutes   _Cook Time:_ 18 minutes
Serves: 4

- 4 (4 oz) turkey tenderloins, about 1/2 inch thick
- 1 tsp ground cumin
- 1/8 tsp black pepper
- 1 Tbsp sugar
- 2 Tbsp vinegar
- 1 1/2 tsp cornstarch
- 1 large tomato, chopped (and seeded if desired)
- 1 cup zucchini, chopped
- 1/4 cup green onions, sliced
- 1 (4 oz) can diced green chili peppers, drained
- 2 cups cooked brown rice

--> Rinse turkey tenderloins and pat dry. Stir together cumin and pepper; sprinkle on both sides of turkey.

--> Spray a large skillet with non-stick cooking spray and heat over medium-high heat. Add turkey and cook both sides until tender and no longer pink. Remove turkey; cover and set aside.

--> For sauce, stir together sugar, vinegar, and cornstarch in a medium bowl. Stir in tomato, zucchini, green onions, and chili peppers. Pour in heated skillet and cook uncovered, on medium-high heat for 5-7 minutes or till mixture is thickened and bubbly, stirring frequently.

--> Spoon over turkey and serve with brown rice.

Grocery List:

4 (4 oz) turkey tenderloins, about 1/2 inch thick
Ground cumin
Sugar
Vinegar
Cornstarch
1 large tomato
1 cup zucchini

Green onions
Brown rice

Per serving _(including rice)_: Calories 285, Total Fat 1g, Sodium 50mg, Carbohydrate 34g, Protein 29g, Fiber 4.3g

MC's Sauteed Shrimp with Peppers

Preparation Time: 15 minutes   _Cooking Time:_ 6 minutes

Serves: 4

- 1 pound shrimp, peeled
- 1 large red pepper, cut into thin strips
- 1 large green pepper, cut into thin strips
- 1/2 cup sliced green onions
- 2 cloves garlic, minced
- 1 cup canned water chestnuts, sliced
- 4 Tbsp apricot preserves
- 2 Tbsp reduced-sodium soy sauce
- 1 tsp toasted sesame seeds
- 2 dashes hot sauce

--> Spray a large skillet with non-stick cooking spray and heat over medium heat. Add red and green peppers, onions, and garlic. Cook for 3-4 minutes or till tender; stirring frequently.

--> Add shrimp and water chestnuts. Cook and stir for 3-4 minutes or till shrimp turn pink. Do not overcook. Remove from heat.

--> Stir in apricot preserves, soy sauce, and hot sauce. Pour mixture over shrimp. Sprinkle with sesame seeds, and serve over brown rice.

Grocery List:

1 pound shrimp, peeled
1 large red pepper
1 large green pepper
Green onions
2 cloves garlic
1 cup canned sliced water chestnuts

Apricot preserves
Reduced-sodium soy sauce
Sesame seeds
Hot sauce
Brown Rice

Per serving: Calories 227, Total Fat 3g, Sodium 43mg, Carbohydrate 30g, Protein 20g, Fiber 2.1g

Tuscan Pork Roast

<u>Preparation Time</u>: 5 minutes   <u>Marinate Time</u>: Overnight
<u>Serves</u>: 10   <u>Cook Time</u>: 1 1/2 hours

- 3 cloves garlic, minced
- 2 Tbsp olive oil
- 1 Tbsp fennel seed, crushed
- 1 Tbsp dried rosemary, crushed
- 1 tsp salt
- 1/4 tsp black pepper
- 1 boneless pork loin roast (about 3 pounds)

--> In a small bowl, combine the first six ingredients and rub over pork. Cover and refrigerate overnight.

--> Place roast on a rack in a shallow roasting pan. Bake at 350°F for 1 1/2 hours or until a meat thermometer reads 160°F. Bast occasionally with pan juices.

--> Let stand 10 minutes before slicing.

Grocery List:
3 cloves garlic
Olive oil
Fennel seed, crushed
Dried rosemary, crushed
1 boneless pork loin roast *(about 3 pounds)*

Per serving: Calories 229 Fat 10g, Sodium 282mg, Carbohydrate 1g, Protein 31g, Fiber 1g

Gingered Pepper Steak

<u>Preparation Time</u>: 10 minutes   <u>Marinate</u>: 2 hours

<u>Serves</u>: 4   <u>Cook Time</u>: 10-15 minutes

- 1/3 reduced-sodium soy sauce
- 2 Tbsp cider vinegar
- 1 Tbsp sugar
- 3/4 tsp ground ginger
- 1 Tbsp cornstarch
- 1 large green pepper, julienned
- 1 large sweet red pepper, julienned
- 1 beef flank steak (about 1 pound), cut in to thin strips
- 1 tsp olive oil

--> Combine soy sauce, vinegar, sugar, and ginger in a small bowl. In a separate small bowl, combine the cornstarch and half of the soy sauce mixture until smooth. Cover and refrigerate.

--> Pour remaining soy sauce mixture into a large resealable plastic bag; add flank steak, seal and turn to coat. Refrigerate for 2 hours.

--> Coat a large wok or non-stick skillet, with cooking spray and heat on medium-high. Add peppers and stir-fry for 3 minutes or until crisp-tender; remove and keep warm.

--> Drain and discard beef marinade. In the same skillet or wok, stir-fry beef in hot oil for 3-4 minutes or until no longer pink.

--> Stir refrigerated soy sauce mixture and pour over beef. Bring to a boil; cook and stir for 2 minutes or until thickened.

--> Return peppers to skillet and heat through. Serve with brown rice if desired.

<u>**Grocery List Next Page**</u>

Gingered Pepper Steak

Grocery List:

Reduced-sodium soy sauce
Apple cider vinegar
Sugar
Ground ginger
Cornstarch
1 large green pepper
1 large sweet red pepper
1 beef flank steak *(about 1 pound)*
Olive oil
Brown rice *(if desired)*

Tip: It's best to choose organic peppers if possible because they absorb more pesticides than most other vegetables.

Per serving: Calories 235, Total Fat 10g, Sodium 875mg, Carbohydrate 12g, Protein 24g, Fiber 2g

Pork and Broccoli Stir-Fry

Preparation Time: 30 minutes   Cooking Time: 8 minutes

Serves: 6

- 1 pound lean boneless pork
- 1 1/2 cup chicken broth
- 1 Tbsp cornstarch
- 4 Tbsp reduced-sodium soy sauce
- 4 Tbsp dry sherry
- 1/4 tsp crushed red pepper
- 2 medium onions, sliced
- 2 (10 oz) packages frozen cut broccoli, thawed and well drained
- 2 cloves garlic, minced
- 1 tsp grated ginger root
- 3 tsp olive oil
- 1 cup canned sliced water chestnuts

--> Partially freeze meat then slice across the grain into bite-size strips.

--> For sauce, stir together chicken broth, cornstarch, soy sauce, dry sherry, and red pepper; set aside.

--> Spray a wok or large skillet with non-stick cooking spray. Add onion, broccoli, garlic, and ginger root and stir-fry for 3-5 minutes or till vegetables are slightly tender. Remove vegetables from skillet.

--> Add olive oil to hot skillet. Add pork and stir-fry for 2-3 minutes or until no longer pink. Push pork to the sides of skillet.

--> Stir sauce and pour in center of skillet. Cook and stir untill thickened and bubbly.

--> Return vegetables to skillet. Add water chestnuts and stir all ingredients together to coat. Cook and stir for 2 minutes more or till heated through.

Grocery List Next Page

Pork and Broccoli Stir-Fry

Grocery List:

1 pound lean boneless pork
Chicken broth
Cornstarch
Reduced-sodium soy sauce
Dry sherry
Crushed red pepper
2 medium onions
2 (10 oz) packages frozen cut broccoli
2 cloves garlic
Ginger root
Olive oil
1 cup canned water chestnuts, sliced

Tip: *If you want to use fresh broccoli instead of frozen, pick out one that is firm and not limp for the best flavor.*

Broccoli is a great vegetable to cook with due to it's high nutrient value. Ounce for ounce, broccoli has more vitamin C than an orange and as much calcium as a glass of milk. It provides a high dose of vitamin A and has three times the fiber of a slice of wheat bran bread.

Per serving: Calories 273, Total Fat 10g, Sodium 933mg, Carbohydrate 18g, Protein 25g, Fiber 3.5g

Spaghetti with Meat Sauce

Preparation Time: 20 minutes   Cooking Time: 35 minutes

Serves: 4

- 1/2 pound extra lean ground turkey or beef
- 1 cup fresh mushrooms, sliced
- 1/2 cup onion, chopped
- 1/2 cup carrot, chopped
- 1/2 cup green pepper, chopped
- 1/4 cup celery, chopped
- 1 clove garlic, minced
- 1 (16 oz) can chopped tomatoes
- 3 oz tomato paste
- 1/4 cup dry red wine
- 1/2 tsp dried basil, crushed
- 1/4 tsp dried oregano, crushed
- 1 small bay leaf
- 1 tsp cornstarch
- 1/4 tsp salt
- 1/8 tsp black pepper
- 6 oz whole wheat spaghetti

--> In a large saucepan cook meat, mushrooms, onion, carrot, green pepper, celery, and garlic till meat is no longer pink and vegetables are tender. Drain any remaining fat.

--> Stir in undrained tomatoes, tomato paste, wine, basil, oregano, bay leaf, salt, and pepper. Bring to boil then reduce heat and cover. Simmer for 30 minutes, stirring occasionally. Remove bay leaf.

--> Combine cornstarch and 1 Tbsp cold water. Stir into sauce. Cook and stir till thickened and bubbly. Cook and stir for 2 minutes more.

--> Meanwhile, cook spaghetti. Drain well and serve with sauce.

Grocery List Next Page

Spaghetti with Meat Sauce

Grocery List:

1/2 pound extra lean ground turkey or beef
1 cup fresh mushrooms
1 onion
Carrots
1 green pepper
Celery
1 clove garlic
1 (16 oz) can chopped tomatoes
3 oz tomato paste
1/4 cup dry red wine or water
Dried basil, crushed
Dried oregano, crushed
Bay leaf
Cornstarch
6 oz whole wheat spaghetti

Tip: *Freeze any leftover red wine you might have so you can use it in the future for recipes such as this. Freezing wine in an ice cube tray makes it easy to measure out the exact amount you need. By doing this, you'll never have to open another bottle just for a recipe and you'll be able to put that last bit of wine that wasn't drunk to good use instead of pouring it out.*

Per serving: Calories 279, Total Fat 3g, Sodium 529mg, Carbohydrate 47g, Protein 20g, Fiber 8.8g

Scallops with Linguine

Preparation Time: **25** minutes   Cook Time: **15–20** minutes

Serves: **6**

- 1 pound fresh or frozen bay scallops
- 12 oz whole wheat linguine
- 1 tsp Smart Balance Butter Spread
- 1 tsp olive oil
- 1 1/2 cups chicken broth
- 3/4 cup dry white wine
- 3 Tbsp lemon juice
- 3/4 cup sliced green onion
- 3/4 cup snipped fresh parsley
- 2 Tbsp capers, drained
- 1 tsp dried dillweed
- 1/4 tsp black pepper

--> Cook linguine according to package directions. Meanwhile, in a large skillet heat Smart Balance and olive oil over medium-high heat. Add scallops; cook and stir about 2 minutes or till opaque. Remove scallops with a slotted spoon, leaving juices in skillet.

--> Stir broth, white wine, and lemon juice into skillet. Bring to a boil and boil for 10–12 minutes or till liquid is reduced to about 1 cup.

--> Stir in onion, parsley, capers, dillweed, and pepper. Reduce heat and simmer uncovered, for about 1 minute.

--> Add scallops, stirring just till heated through. Pour over pasta; toss gently.

Grocery List Next Page

Scallops with Linguine

Grocery List:

1 pound fresh or frozen bay scallops
12 oz whole wheat linguine
Smart Balance Butter Spread
Olive oil
Chicken broth
White wine
Lemon juice
Green onion
Fresh parsley
Capers
Dried dillweed

Tip: *You can substitute sea scallops for the bay scallops if you prefer. Bay scallops however, tend to be sweeter than sea scallops and are usually cheaper.*

Per serving: Calories 320, Total Fat 5g, Sodium 305mg, Carbohydrate 50g, Protein 21g, Fiber 7g

Shrimp and Broccoli Stir-Fry with Peppers

Preparation Time: 15 minutes   Cook Time: 15 minutes

Serves: 4

- 2 Tbsp reduced-sodium soy sauce (divided)
- 1 Tbsp rice vinegar or sherry
- 1 1/2 Tbsp cornstarch (divided)
- 3/4 pound medium shrimp, peeled and deveined
- 3/4 cup chicken broth (reduced-sodium)
- 1 tsp sugar
- 2 Tbsp olive oil
- 3 cloves garlic, minced
- 1 Tbsp ginger, finely chopped
- 1 stalk celery, sliced diagonally
- 2 cups broccoli florets
- 1 sweet red pepper, cut into strips
- 1 1/2 cups sugar snapped peas, trimmed

--> Combine 1 Tbsp soy sauce, rice vinegar, and 1/2 Tbsp cornstarch in a bowl. Stir in shrimp; cover, and marinate about 15 minutes.

--> In another bowl, combine 1/4 cup chicken broth with remaining soy sauce, cornstarch, and sugar.

--> Heat 1 Tbsp olive oil in wok or large skillet. Add garlic and ginger; stir-fry about 30 seconds. Add celery, broccoli, and pepper, and stir-fry about 2 minutes. Stir in remaining chicken broth; reduce heat, cover and cook about 3 minutes.

--> Add peas; cover and cook about 2 minutes longer or until vegetables are tender.

--> Stir in cornstarch mixture and cook, stirring constantly, about 1 minute. Stir in shrimp and cook about 1 minute longer or until just heated through.

Grocery List Next Page

Shrimp and Broccoli Stir-Fry with Peppers

Grocery List:

Reduced-sodium soy sauce
Rice vinegar or sherry
Cornstarch
3/4 pound medium shrimp
Chicken broth (reduced-sodium)
Sugar
Olive oil
3 cloves garlic, minced
Ginger, finely chopped
Celery
2 cups broccoli florets
1 sweet red pepper
1 1/2 cups sugar snapped peas

Tip: Shrimp can be a dieter's dream since it only has 90 calories and 1.5 grams of fat per 3 ounce serving. Always try to buy U.S. shrimp because it has the best flavor.

Per serving: Calories 208, Total Fat 8g, Sodium 431mg, Carbohydrate 16g, Protein 17g, Fiber 3g

Spinach and Chicken Turnovers

<u>Preparation Time:</u> 18 minutes   <u>Cook Time:</u> 20 minutes

<u>Serves:</u> 4

- 1 cup finely chopped cooked chicken or turkey
- 1/2 of a 10 oz pkg frozen chopped spinach, thawed and well drained
- 1/3 cup shredded low-fat mozzarella cheese
- 3 Tbsp sliced green onion
- 1/2 tsp dried oregano, crushed
- 1/8 tsp garlic salt
- Dash black pepper
- 3/4 cup Heart Healthy Biscuit Mix
- 1/2 cup whole wheat flour
- 1/3 cup skim milk
- 1/2 cup pizza sauce

--> For filling, combine chicken, spinach, cheese, onion, oregano, garlic salt, and pepper in a mixing bowl, set aside.

--> In a separate bowl, stir together biscuit mix and flour. Stir in milk just till moistened. Turn dough out onto a lightly floured surface and knead 10-12 strokes. Divide dough into 4 equal pieces. Roll each piece into a 7-inch circle.

--> Spoon 1/4 of the filling onto one half of each circle of dough. Fold the other half of the dough over the filling and seal edges with the tines of a fork. Place turnovers on an ungreased baking sheet.

--> Bake at 400°F for about 20 minutes or till golden. Meanwhile, in a small saucepan, heat pizza sauce. Serve with hot turnovers.

Grocery List Next Page

Spinach and Chicken Turnovers

Grocery List:
1 cup finely chopped cooked chicken or turkey
5 oz frozen spinach
1/3 cup shredded low-fat mozzarella cheese
Green onions
Dried oregano, crushed
Garlic salt
Heart Healthy Biscuit Mix
Whole wheat flour
Skim milk
Pizza sauce

Tip: I recommended the Heart Healty Biscuit Mix over the original mix because it doesn't contain trans fats. I was so excited when they came up with the Heart Healthy Mix because I wouldn't cook with the original since it contained partially hydrogenated oil.

Per serving: Calories 285, Total Fat 8g, Sodium 631mg, Carbohydrate 32g, Protein 21g, Fiber 6.4g

Eggplant Parmesan

Preparation Time: 15 minutes   Cook Time: 50 minutes

Serves: 4

- 1 egg, beaten
- 1/4 cup skim milk
- 1/8 tsp black pepper
- 1 cup reduced sodium saltine crackers, crushed (about 28 crackers)
- 1/4 cup grated Parmesan cheese
- 2 Tbsp dried parsley flakes
- 1 medium eggplant, sliced 1/4 inch thick (about 1 pound)
- 1 (15 oz) can seasoned tomato sauce
- 1/2 tsp dried oregano, crushed
- 1 clove garlic, minced
- 3/4 cup shredded part-skim mozzarella cheese (3 oz)

--> In a small bowl combine egg, milk, and pepper. In another bowl stir together cracker crumbs, Parmesan cheese, and dried parsley flakes.

--> Dip eggplant slices in the milk mixture to coat, then dip in cracker mixture making sure to completely coat both sides.

--> Arrange eggplant on a baking dish that has been coated with a non-stick cooking spray.

--> In a bowl stir together tomato sauce, oregano, and garlic; pour over eggplant.

--> Cover and bake for 40 minutes at 350°F or till eggplant is tender. Sprinkle with mozzarella cheese and continue to bake uncovered, 10 minutes more.

Grocery List Next Page

Eggplant Parmesan

Grocery List:
1 egg
Skim milk
Reduced sodium saltine crackers
Grated Parmesan cheese
Dried parsley flakes
1 medium eggplant
1 (15 oz) can seasoned tomato sauce
Dried oregano, crushed
1 clove garlic
3/4 cup shredded part-skim mozzarella cheese (3 oz)

Tip: *Eggplants are the best when in season from August to October. When picking an eggplant, choose the ones that are small to medium sized for the best flavor.*

This vegetable is a dieter's true friend because of its high fiber content that will not only make you feel fuller longer, but also aid you in your digestive function and lower your risk of coronary diesease.

Per serving: Calories 249, Total Fat 9g, Sodium 900mg, Carbohydrate 28g, Protein 15g, Fiber 6.4g

Tofu and Vegetable Stir-Fry

Preparation Time: 15 minutes   _Cook Time:_ 8 minutes

Serves: 4

- 1 cup water
- 1/2 cup dry sherry
- 2 Tbsp cornstarch
- 4 Tbsp reduced sodium soy sauce
- 2 tsp sugar
- 2 tsp instant chicken bouillon granules
- 1 1/2 tsp ground ginger
- 2 cups carrots, thinly sliced
- 2 garlic cloves, minced
- 6 cups broccoli, cut-up
- 12 oz extra-firm tofu, cubed
- 2 Tbsp toasted sesame seeds
- 2 cups brown rice, cooked

--> Stir together water, dry sherry, cornstarch, soy sauce, sugar, bouillon granules, and ginger, set aside.

--> Spray a wok or non-stick skillet with non-stick cooking spray and preheat over medium-high heat. Add carrots and garlic and stir-fry for 2 minutes. Add broccoli and stir-fry for 3-4 minutes or till all vegetables are crisp-tender. Push vegetables to the side of wok or skillet.

--> Stir sauce and add to the center of skillet. Cook and stir till thickened and bubbly. Add tofu and stir together to coat with sauce. Cook and stir for 1 minute.

--> Serve over hot cooked brown rice. Sprinkle with sesame seeds.

Grocery List Next Page

Tofu and Vegetable Stir-Fry

Grocery List:
Dry sherry
Cornstarch
Reduced sodium soy sauce
Sugar
Instant chicken bouillon granules
Ground ginger
Carrots
2 garlic cloves, minced
Broccoli
12 oz extra-firm tofu
Toasted sesame seeds
Brown rice

Tip: To toast sesame seeds, just heat a dab of olive oil in a skillet and add the seeds, Stir frequently until they're a light golden brown. You can also spray the skillet with non-stick cooking spray if you want to leave out the fat from the oil.

Per serving *(including rice)*:
Calories 325, Total Fat 5g,
Sodium 729mg, Carbohydrate 51g,
Protein 15g, Fiber 7.8g

VEGETABLES & SIDE DISHES

Stir-Fried Broccoli with Sesame Seeds

Preparation Time: **3 minutes**   Cook Time: **8-10 Minutes**
Serves: **4**

- 1 Tbsp sesame seeds
- 1/2 Tbsp extra virgin olive oil
- 1 Tbsp reduced-sodium soy sauce
- 1/8 tsp hot red pepper flakes
- 1 bunch broccoli, cut stalks and reserve florets
- 1/4 cup water
- 1/8 tsp salt
- 1/8 tsp pepper

--> Heat a large non-stick skillet. Add sesame seeds and toast, shaking pan constantly, 1-2 minutes or until seeds turn golden.

--> Remove skillet from heat and transfer seeds to a plate. Return skillet to heat, add oil, soy sauce, and hot red pepper flakes, stir to combine.

--> Add broccoli florets and stir-fry about 2 minutes. Add water and cover skillet.

--> Cook broccoli 1-2 minutes longer or until crisp-tender.

--> Stir in sesame seeds and season with salt and pepper.

Grocery List:
Sesame seeds
Extra virgin olive oil
Reduced-sodium soy sauce
Hot red pepper flakes
1 bunch broccoli

Per serving: Calories 46, Total Fat 4g,
Sodium 196mg, Carbohydrate 24g,
Protein 6g, Fiber 5g

Steamed Broccoli

<u>Preparation Time:</u> 5 minutes   <u>Cook Time:</u> 4-5 minutes
<u>Serves:</u> 4

- 1 bunch fresh broccoli, cut into spears
- 1 tsp olive oil
- 1/8 tsp salt

--> Wash broccoli, place in a microwavable dish, and sprinkle
with salt and olive oil.

--> Cover and microwave on high for 2-3 minutes; stir and
cook for 2-3 minutes more or until broccoli can be pierced
with a fork. Do not overcook. Times will vary depending on
the wattage of your microwave.

Grocery List:
Broccoli
Olive oil

Tip: Fresh broccoli tastes so much better than broccoli that
has started to age. Try to time your recipes so that you purchase
and cook broccoli the same or the following day to get the best
flavor. Using fresh broccoli will also increase the odds that your
children will eat it.

Per serving: Calories 70 , Total Fat 2.8g,
Sodium 123mg, Carbohydrate 10g,
Protein 4.3g, Fiber 4g

Steamed Asparagus

Preparation Time: 2 minutes   Cook Time: 2-4 minutes
Serves: 4

- 20 stalks of fresh asparagus
- 1/2 tsp olive oil
- 1/8 tsp salt

--> Cut off and discard bottom 1/3 of asparagus and wash. Pat dry; brush on olive oil.

--> Place in a microwave-proof shallow dish and add 1 Tbsp of water and cover.

--> Sprinkle with salt and cook on high for about 2-4 minutes depending on the wattage of your microwave. Do not overcook.

Grocery List:
1 pound fresh asparagus
Olive oil

Tip: Dieters love asparagus because it's a natural diuretic. Take advantage of this benefit by eating asparagus around your menstrual cycle to help reduce bloating.

Per serving: Calories 40, Total Fat 1.75g, Sodium 74mg, Carbohydrate 0g, Protein .5g, Fiber .5g

Sauteed Squash and Zucchini

Preparation Time: 5 minutes   Cook Time: 12-14 Minutes
Serves: 6

- 1 Tbsp olive oil
- 2 medium yellow squash, sliced
- 2 medium zucchini, sliced
- 2 garlic cloves, finely chopped
- 1 Tbsp fresh oregano
- 1/8 tsp salt and black pepper to taste

--> Heat oil in a large skillet over medium-high heat and add garlic; cook 3 minutes.

--> Add squash and zucchini and cook, stirring occasionally, until golden brown or about 10-12 minutes.

--> Stir in oregano, salt and black pepper and cook for 2 more minutes. Serve immediately.

Grocery List:

Olive oil
2 medium yellow squash
2 medium zucchini
Fresh oregano
Garlic

Tip: Pick out squash that is small to medium for the best flavor. You also want squash that is firm and not soft.

Per serving: Calories 41, Total Fat 2.6g, Sodium 49mg, Carbohydrate 2.6g, Protein 1.5g, Fiber 1.6g

Simple Sauteed Mushrooms and Onions

Preparation Time: 5 minutes   Cook Time: 8-10 Minutes

Serves: 4

- 8 oz whole mushrooms, sliced
- 1 medium sweet onion, chopped
- 1/2 Tbsp olive oil
- 1 Tbsp Worcestershire Sauce
- 1/4 tsp garlic powder
- Salt and pepper to taste

--> Heat olive oil in a medium skillet over medium-high heat. Add onions and cook 1-2 minutes, stirring frequently.

--> Add mushrooms, Worcestershire Sauce, and garlic powder. Stir frequently and cook for about 7-8 minutes or until desired tenderness. Add salt and pepper to taste.

Grocery List:
8 oz whole mushrooms
1 medium sweet onion
Olive oil
Worcestershire Sauce
Garlic powder

Per serving: Calories 62, Total Fat 2.2g, Sodium 55mg, Carbohydrate 8g, Protein 4.3g, Fiber 2g

Broccoli and Pasta with Onion Sauce

Preparation Time: 10 minutes   Cooking Time: 15 minutes
Serves: 4-6

- 3 oz whole wheat linguine or fettuccine
- 1 1/2 cups fresh broccoli florets
- 1 medium sweet onion, sliced and separated into rings
- 3/4 cup skim milk
- 2 tsp cornstarch
- 1 tsp instant chicken bouillon granules
- 2 Tbsp dry white wine
- 2 oz shredded part-skim mozzarella cheese
- Dash black pepper
- Dash ground nutmeg

--> Cook pasta according to package directions, adding broccoli during the last 5 minutes of cooking. Drain well.

--> Meanwhile, spray a large skillet with non-stick cooking spray and add onions. Cook, covered, over medium-low heat for about 10 minutes or till onions are tender, stirring occasionally.

--> In a small bowl stir together milk, cornstarch, bouillon granules, black pepper, and nutmeg. Add mixture to onion in skillet. Cook and stir over medium heat till thickened and bubbly. Once thickened, cook for 2 minutes more.

--> Stir in wine and cheese till cheese is melted. Pour cheese mixture over pasta and broccoli; toss to coat and serve.

Grocery List:

Whole wheat linguine or fettuccine
Broccoli
1 sweet onion
Skim milk
Cornstarch
Instant chicken bouillon granules
Dry white wine

2 oz shredded part-skim
   mozzarella cheese
Ground nutmeg

Per serving: Calories 132, Total Fat 3g, Sodium 161mg, Carbohydrate 19g, Protein 7g, Fiber 2.1g

Fluffy Dilled Carrots and Potatoes

<u>Preparation Time:</u> 15 minutes   <u>Cook Time:</u> 15 minutes
<u>Serves:</u> 4

- 1 1/2 cups sliced carrots
- 3/4 cup peeled and sliced red potato
- 1 1/2 Tbsp skim milk
- 2 tsp Smart Balance Butter Spread
- 1/4 tsp salt
- 1/4 tsp dried dillweed
- 1/4 – 1/8 tsp onion powder
- Dash black pepper

--> Combine carrots, potato, and 1/2 cup water in a 1 1/2 quart microwave-safe casserole dish. Cook in microwave, covered, on high for 10-12 minutes or until very tender, stirring once. Drain.

--> Mash vegetables and add milk, butter, salt, dillweed, onion powder, and pepper. Beat or mash until nearly smooth.

--> Return mixture to casserole dish, cover and cook on high for 1-2 minutes or till heated through.

Grocery List:
Carrots
Red potatoes
Skim milk
Smart Balance Butter Spread
Dried dillweed
Onion powder

Per serving: Calories 86, Total Fat 3g, Sodium 238mg, Carbohydrate 15g, Protein 2g, Fiber 2.1g

Baked Onion Rings

Preparation Time: 3 minutes   Cook Time: 15 - 18 minutes
Serves: 4

- 1/2 cup egg substitute
- 2/3 cup dry bread crumbs (plain or seasoned)
- 1/2 tsp salt
- 1/4 tsp pepper
- 1 sweet onion, sliced and separated into rings

--> Place egg substitute in a shallow dish. In another shallow dish, combine the bread crumbs, salt and pepper.

--> Dip onion rings into egg, then roll in crumb mixture.

--> Spray a baking sheet with nonstick cooking spray and place onion rings in a single layer.

--> Bake at 425°F for 15-18 minutes or until golden brown, turning once half way through cooking time.

Grocery List:
Egg substitute
Dry bread crumbs (plain or seasoned)
1 sweet onion

Tip: We tend to forget about the nutritional value of the commonly used onion. Onions can reduce the risk of certain types of cancer and diabetes, boost your HDL (or good cholesterol), and attack bacteria that can cause infection.

Per serving: Calories 66, Total Fat 1g, Sodium 312mg, Carbohydrate 12g, Protein 3g, Fiber 1g

Summer Squash Medley

Preparation Time: 10 minutes   Cook Time: 10 minutes
Serves: 6

- 3 medium yellow squash, sliced
- 2 medium zucchini, sliced
- 1 medium red onion, sliced and separated into rings
- 1 tsp minced garlic
- 1 Tbsp olive oil
- 1 tsp dried parsley flakes
- 1 tsp dried basil
- 1 tsp dried oregano
- 1/2 tsp dried thyme
- 1/4 tsp salt
- 1/2 cup part-skim mozzarella cheese, shredded

--> Heat oil in a large skillet. Saute yellow squash, zucchini, onion, and garlic until crisp-tender, stirring occasionally.

--> Stir in parsley, basil, oregano, thyme, and salt. Remove from heat and transfer to a serving dish.

--> Sprinkle with cheese; cover and let stand until cheese is melted.

Grocery List:
3 medium yellow squash
2 medium zucchini
1 medium red onion
Garlic
Olive oil
Dried parsley flakes
Dried basil
Dried oregano
Dried thyme
1/2 cup part-skim mozzarella cheese, shredded

Per serving: Calories 83, Total Fat 4g,
Sodium 147mg, Carbohydrate 9g,
Protein 5g, Fiber 3g

Stir-Fried Carrots

Preparation Time: 5 minutes   Cook Time: 10-12 minutes
Serves: 4

- 1 1/2 pounds fresh carrots, julienned
- 1 Tbsp olive oil
- 1/2 cup chicken broth (reduced sodium)
- 1 tsp dried rosemary, crushed
- 1/4 tsp black pepper

--> Heat olive oil in a large skillet or wok. Add carrots and stir-fry until crisp-tender.

--> Stir in broth, rosemary, and pepper and bring to a boil.

--> Reduce heat; simmer, uncovered until liquid is reduced, about 2-3 minutes.

Grocery List:

Carrots
Olive oil
Chicken broth (reduced sodium)
Dried rosemary, crushed

Tip: *Yes, it's true! Carrots are good for your eyes. They are an excellent source of antioxidant compounds including beta-carotene which protects your vision, especially night vision. It also protects your eyes from macular degeneration and the development of senile cataracts – the two leading causes of blindness in the elderly.*
See, Mom was right!

Per serving: Calories 106, Total Fat 4g, Sodium 70mg, Carbohydrate 18g, Protein 2g, Fiber 5g

Seasoned Brown Rice

<u>Preparation Time:</u> 5 minutes   <u>Cook Time:</u> 40 - 45 minutes
<u>Serves:</u> 4

- 1 1/3 cups water
- 2/3 cup long grain brown rice
- 1 Tbsp reduced sodium soy sauce
- 1/2 tsp dried basil
- 1/4 - 1/2 tsp ground ginger
- 1/8 tsp cayenne pepper

--> In a small saucepan, bring water and rice to a boil.
--> Reduce heat and cover. Simmer for 35-45 minutes or until water is absorbed and rice is tender.
--> Stir in remaining ingredients.

Grocery List:

Long grain brown rice
Reduced sodium soy sauce
Dried basil
Ground ginger
Cayenne pepper

Tip: Brown rice has almost 6 times the amount of fiber than white rice. If you haven't made the switch to brown rice yet, now is the time to do. Choosing brown rice over white will help you with your weight loss and improve your overall health.

Per serving: Calories 118, Total Fat 1g, Sodium 157mg, Carbohydrate 24g, Protein 3g, Fiber 2g

Gready's Stir-Fry Cabbage

<u>Preparation Time:</u> 5 minutes   <u>Cook Time:</u> 5 - 7 minutes

<u>Serves:</u> 4 - 6

- 2 Tbsp olive oil
- 2 cloves garlic, minced
- 1 small sweet onion, sliced into thin strips
- 1 head cabbage, sliced on an angle into thin strips
- 1 tsp Nature's Seasoning

--> Heat oil and add onion and garlic. Add cabbage and stir frequently over medium heat until cabbage is cooked down and soft.

--> Serve with hot pepper vinegar.

Grocery List:
Olive oil
Garlic
1 small sweet onion
1 head cabbage
Nature's Seasoning

Tip: Cabbage is another great diet food because one cup of shredded cabbage is only 17 calories yet it's packed with vitamins A, C, E and B.

Per serving: Calories 102, Total Fat 5.9g, Sodium 41mg, Carbohydrate 12g, Protein 2.8g, Fiber 4.4g

Baked Sweet Potato Sticks

Preparation Time: 5 minutes   _Cook Time:_ 40 minutes
Serves: 6

- 6 small sweet potatoes
- 1 Tbsp olive oil
- 1/2 tsp paprika

--> Slice potatoes lengthwise into sticks.

--> Mix together oil and paprika. Add potato sticks and coat completely. Spray a baking sheet with non-stick cooking spray and place potato sticks, in a single layer.

--> Bake at 400°F for about 40 minutes or till desired crispness.

Grocery List:
6 small sweet potatoes
Olive oil
Paprika

Tip: Leave the skin on sweet potatoes to maximize their nutritional value.

Per serving: Calories 100, Total Fat 2.5g,
Sodium 55mg, Carbohydrate 19g,
Protein 1.4g, Fiber 2.8g

DESSERTS

Fresh Fruit and Dip

Preparation Time: 10 minutes   Cook Time: 0
Serves: 6

- 8 oz carton plain low-fat yogurt
- 1/4 cup unsweetened applesauce
- 1/2 tsp vanilla
- 1/8 tsp ground cinnamon
- 1 Tbsp powdered sugar
- 3 cups assorted sliced fresh fruit (such as pineapple chunks, strawberries, apple slices, and peach slices)

--> In a small bowl stir together yogurt, applesauce, powdered sugar, vanilla, and cinnamon.
--> Spoon fruit into individual bowls, top with dip and serve.

Grocery List:
8 oz carton plain low-fat yogurt
Unsweetened applesauce
Vanilla extract
Ground cinnamon
Powdered sugar
3 cups assorted sliced fresh fruit
   (such as pineapple chunks, strawberries, apple slices, and peach slices)

Per serving: Calories 87, Total Fat 1g, Sodium 28mg, Carbohydrate 18g, Protein 3g, Fiber 2g

Easy Strawberry Shortcakes

Preparation: **3** minutes   Cook Time: **0** minutes
Serves: **4**   Freeze Time: **8** hours

- 4 (1 oz) slices of angel food cake
- 2 cups fresh, sliced strawberries; place in a plastic airtight bag and put in freezer for 6-8 hours and then thaw to create a sugar-free syrup (if you're short on time you may use a 16 oz package frozen sliced strawberries, in a light syrup)
- Whipped topping

--> Place sliced angel food cake on a plate and cover with
    V4 cup of strawberries with its own syrup.
--> Top with V4 cup whipped topping and serve.

Grocery List:

Angel food cake
Fresh strawberries or 16 oz frozen
Whipped topping

Tip: Strawberries are one of the fruits that should be purchased organic if possible. They, along with blueberries and peaches, tend to absorb high amounts of pesticides and other chemicals. If you can't buy organic strawberries, buy the ones that are grown in the U.S. Our government regulates the chemicals used in farming so our produce tends to have lower levels of pesticide than other countries where they don't have strict regulations.

Per serving: Calories 105, Total Fat .4g,
Sodium 155mg, Carbohydrate 25g,
Protein 2.5g, Fiber 3g

Rhubarb and Strawberry Sauce

Preparation Time: 10 minutes   Cook Time: 8 minutes

Serves: 6   Chill Time: 1 1/2 hours

- 1/4 cup sugar
- 1/4 cup orange juice
- 2 cups rhubarb cut into 1/2" slices or 8 oz frozen sliced rhubarb
- 2 tsp cornstarch
- 1 Tbsp water
- 1 cup fresh strawberries, sliced

--> Combine sugar and orange juice in a small saucepan. Bring to a boil then add rhubarb. Return to boil then reduce heat. Cover and simmer for 5-7 minutes or until rhubarb is nearly tender.

--> Drain rhubarb, reserving liquid. Add water to syrup to make 2/3 cup.

--> Stir together cornstarch and water; stir into syrup, cook and stir until thickened and bubbly. Cook and stir for 2 minutes more. Remove saucepan from heat.

--> Gently stir in rhubarb and strawberries. Cover and chill thoroughly - about 1 1/2 hours.

Grocery List:

Sugar
Orange juice
2 cups rhubarb or 8 oz frozen sliced rhubarb
Cornstarch
Fresh strawberries

Per serving: Calories 61, Total Fat .5g, Sodium 5mg, Carbohydrate 15g, Protein 1g, Fiber 1.5g

Watermelon and Strawberry Sorbet

Preparation Time: 15 minutes   Chill Time: 3 hours
Serves: 6

- 1/2 cup sugar
- 1 cup water
- 2 cups seedless watermelon, cubed
- 2 cups fresh strawberries, hulled
- 1 Tbsp fresh mint, minced
- Mint leaves for garnish if desired

--> In a small heavy saucepan, bring the water and sugar to a boil. Cook and stir until sugar is dissolved. Remove from heat and allow to slightly cool.

--> Put watermelon and strawberries in a blender and add the sugar syrup. Process for 3 minutes or until smooth. Strain and discard any seeds and pulp.

--> Transfer puree to a 13 x 9 x 2" dish. Freeze for 1 hour or until the edges begin to firm.

--> Stir in mint and freeze 2 more hours or until firm. Right before serving, place mixture in a blender and process for 3 minutes or until smooth. Transfer to serving bowls and garnish with mint leaves if desired.

Grocery List:

Sugar
Watermelon
2 cups fresh strawberries
Fresh mint
Mint leaves for garnish if desired

Per serving: Calories 95, Total Fat .5g,
Sodium 3mg, Carbohydrate 25g,
Protein 1g, Fiber 2g

Peach Cobbler

<u>Preparation Time:</u> 15 minutes   <u>Cook Time:</u> 25-30 minutes

<u>Serves:</u> 6

- 1/4 cup water
- 1/4 cup peach or apricot preserves
- 1 Tbsp cornstarch
- 1 tsp lemon juice
- 2 cups frozen peaches, thawed and cubed

<u>Topping:</u>
- 1/3 cup whole wheat flour
- 1/3 cup all-purpose flour
- 1/4 cup rolled oats
- 2 Tbsp brown sugar
- 1 tsp baking powder
- 1/4 tsp ground cinnamon
- 1 egg
- 1/4 cup low-fat milk

--> In a medium saucepan, combine water, preserves, cornstarch and lemon juice; stir until blended. Stir in peaches and cook over medium-low heat for about 5 minutes; stir constantly until the mixture boils and thickens. Let boil for 1 minute, stirring constantly. Remove from heat and cover to keep warm.

--> To make topping; combine flour, oats, brown sugar, baking powder and cinnamon in a medium mixing bowl. In a separate small bowl, mix milk and egg together and add to the flour mixture. Mix until it forms a soft, spoonable dough.

--> Transfer the peach mixture to a lightly greased 8 x 8 x 2" baking dish. Using a spoon, drop small portions of the dough over the peaches to make a "cobbled" effect.

--> Bake 20-30 minutes at 400°F or until bubbling, crisp, and golden.

Peach Cobbler

Grocery List:
Peach or apricot preserves
Cornstarch
Lemon juice
2 cups frozen peaches

Topping:
Whole-wheat flour
All-purpose flour
Rolled oats
2 Tbsp brown sugar
Baking powder
Ground cinnamon
1 egg
Low-fat milk

Tip: This dessert is great served with a bowl of frozen low-fat vanilla yogurt!

Per serving: Calories 190, Total Fat 1g,
Sodium 71mg, Carbohydrate 42g,
Protein 4g, Fiber 3g

Blueberry Oat Crisp

<u>Preparation Time:</u> 15 minutes   <u>Cook Time:</u> 25-30 minutes

<u>Serves:</u> 6

- 1/4 cup blueberry preserves
- 1 Tbsp cornstarch
- 1 tsp lemon juice
- 1/8 tsp ground nutmeg
- 4 cups blueberries, fresh or frozen and thawed

<u>Topping:</u> (same as Peach Cobbler recipe)
- 1/3 cup whole wheat flour
- 1/3 cup all-purpose flour
- 1/4 cup rolled oats
- 2 Tbsp brown sugar
- 1 tsp baking powder
- 1/4 tsp ground cinnamon
- 1 egg
- 1/4 cup low-fat milk

--> In a saucepan, combine preserves, cornstarch, lemon juice, and nutmeg. Stir until blended. Stir in blueberries and cook over moderate heat for about 5 minutes; stir constantly until the the mixture boils and thickens. Boil for 1 minute, stirring constantly. Remove from heat and keep warm.

--> To make topping; combine flour, oats, brown sugar, baking powder and cinnamon in a medium mixing bowl. In a separate small bowl, mix milk and egg together and add to flour mixture. Mix until it forms a soft, spoonable dough.

--> Transfer filling into a lightly greased 8 x 8 x 2" baking dish and use a spoon to drop small portions of the dough over the blueberry mixture to form a "cobbled" effect.

--> Bake at 400°F for 20-25 minutes or until bubbling and crisp.

Blueberry Oat Crisp

Grocery List:
Blueberry preserves
Cornstarch
Lemon juice
Ground nutmeg
4 cups blueberries, fresh or frozen
Whole wheat flour
All-purpose flour
Rolled oats
Brown sugar
Baking powder
Ground cinnamon
1 egg
Low-fat milk

Tip: If you want to work ahead, you can mix the first 6 ingredients of the topping a few days in advance. Store in an airtight container until you're ready to use it.

Per serving: Calories 189, Total Fat 2g, Sodium 78mg, Carbohydrate 41g, Protein 4g, Fiber 4g

www.ingramcontent.com/pod-product-compliance
Lightning Source LLC
Chambersburg PA
CBHW051957280526
45793CB00005B/753